Accession no.
01148409

W
18.7.05

Sexuality, Sexual Health and Ageing

D0318072

Sexuality, Sexual Health and Ageing

Merryn Gott

Open University Press

Open University Press
McGraw-Hill Education
McGraw-Hill House
Shoppenhangers Road
Maidenhead, Berkshire
England SL6 2QL

email: enquiries@openup.co.uk
world wide web: www.openup.co.uk

and Two Penn Plaza, New York, NY 10121–2289, USA

First published 2005

Copyright © Merryn Gott 2005

All rights reserved. Except for the quotation of short passages for the purpose of
criticism and review, no part of this publication may be reproduced, stored in a
retrieval system, or transmitted, in any form or by any means, electronic, mechanical,
photocopying, recording or otherwise, without the prior written permission of the
publisher or a licence from the Copyright Licensing Agency Limited. Details of such
licences (for reprographic reproduction) may be obtained from the Copyright Licensing
Agency Ltd of 90 Tottenham Court Road, London, W1T 4LP.

A catalogue record of this book is available from the British Library

ISBN 0 335 21018 X (pb)   0 335 21019 8 (hb)

Library of Congress Cataloging-in-Publication Data
CIP data has been applied for

Typeset by BookEns Ltd, Royston, Herts.
Printed and bound in Great Britain by
MPG Books Ltd, Bodmin, Cornwall

Contents

Series editor's preface

Sexuality, Sexual Health and Ageing by Merryn Gott is the twentieth book to be published in the *Rethinking Ageing* series and it seems appropriate to locate it in the context of what has been achieved. The series was planned in the early 1990s, following the rapid growth in ageing populations in Britain and other countries that led to a dramatic increase in academic and professional interest in gerontology. In the 1970s and 80s there was a steady increase in the publication of research studies which defined the characteristics and needs of older people. There were also a small number of theoretical attempts to re-conceptualise the meaning of old age and to explore new ways in which we could think about ageing. By the early 1990s, however, a palpable gap had emerged between what was known about ageing by gerontologists and the very limited amount of information which was readily available to the growing number of people with a professional or personal interest in old age. The *Rethinking Ageing* series was conceived as a response to that 'knowledge gap'.

The first book to be published in the new series was *Age, Race and Ethnicity* by Ken Blakemore and Margaret Boneham. In the series editor's preface I set out the main aim of the *Rethinking Ageing* series which was to focus on a topic of current concern or interest in ageing by addressing two fundamental questions: what is known about this topic? and, what are the policy and practice implications of this knowledge? We wanted authors to provide a readable and stimulating review of current knowledge, but also to *rethink* their subject area by developing their own ideas in the light of their particular research and experience. We also believed it was essential that the books should be both scholarly *and* written in clear, non-technical, language that would appeal equally to a broad range of students, academics and professionals with a common interest in ageing and age care.

The books published in this series have ranged broadly in subject matter, including policy and practice in health and community care, ageism, reminiscence, residential care, the politics of later life, and dementia. We have been very pleased that the response by readers and reviewers has been extremely positive to almost all of the titles and that some have had a profound influence on thought and practice – for example, Tom Kitwood's

Dementia Reconsidered is widely regarded as a seminal text. The success of the series appears therefore to have justified its original aims.

Now, well over a decade later, age is a prominent topic in media and government policy debates. This reflects a new awareness of the demographic situation. However, although there is more interest in ageing and old age than when we started the *Rethinking Ageing* series, we believe there is still a need for the serious but accessible, topic-based books about ageing that it offers. Moreover, having addressed many of the staple topics of gerontology, we felt five years ago that it was time for the series to extend its subject-matter to include emerging topics and those whose importance were yet to be widely appreciated. Among the first books to reflect this policy were Maureen Crane's *Understanding Older Homeless People* and John Vincent's *Politics, Power and Old Age*. More recently, Mike Hepworth's *Stories of Ageing* was the first book by an author based in the UK to explore the potential of literary fiction as a gerontological resource. At the same time, we have continued to include topics of established interest as reflected in 2002 in *Housing and Home in Later Life* by Frances Heywood, Christine Oldman and Robin Means, and earlier this year, *Quality of Life* by John Bond and Lynne Corner.

As the twentieth book in the series we are very happy to publish a ground-breaking study of sexuality, sexual health and ageing. Not only does Merryn Gott address a topic which even today is seldom discussed, she does so by questioning both the traditional view that older people are asexual and the new myth of what she calls the 'sexy oldie', suggesting that the latter may be equally as oppressive as the former. Focusing upon studies of older people's experience, she raises important questions such as: what do we know about sexuality and ageing? How important is sex to older people? And how do people differ in respect of later life sexuality?

Gott examines the social framework of sexuality in relation to ageing and argues that sexuality does not have to have just one meaning. For example, she suggests that prevalent definitions of sexuality may be too narrow with rates of sexual intercourse being regarded as the only measure of sexual activity and other forms of sexuality being disregarded. In questioning too the wisdom of the new social emphasis on the responsibility of the ageing person to remain sexual (rather than regarding this as a choice), Gott opens up an important area for debate and makes a strong case for viewing sexuality within the totality of later life experience.

As the title of her book suggests, Gott also examines sexual health and sexual problems drawing on empirical studies including her own research. Among the key questions she addresses are: what is sexual health? What is the extent of sexual 'dysfunction' among older people? What is the impact of sexual problems on older individuals and upon sexual relationships? And what are older people's experiences of seeking treatment for sexual problems? In the final chapter she considers the health professional's role in later life sexuality and makes recommendations concerning sexual health management.

This is a deeply considered and lucidly argued book which questions our assumptions on an important topic and presents new evidence. It will move forward the debate on sexuality in later life and is an excellent addition to the *Rethinking Ageing* series.

Brian Gearing

School of Health and Social Welfare
The Open University

Acknowledgements

I would like to thank Kevin Morgan for convincing me it was a good idea to write this book (I now believe him). Thanks also for useful comments on early drafts.

Thank you to Sharron Hinchliff who has played an integral role in much of the original research presented in this book, and Kate Chadwick for her help in preparing the manuscript.

Thank you to everyone at Open University Press and, particularly, Rachel Gear, for her patience.

Finally, thank you to my family, for everything.

Introduction

Sex and sexuality have become preoccupations of modern society. We live in a 'sexualized world' (Hawkes 1996: 1), constantly bombarded by sexual imagery and language. Sex has becomes more visible in the literature we read, the films and television programmes we watch, and is used to sell us everything from razors to holidays. Books and manuals exist advising us on all aspects of sexuality, from how to be sexually attractive to more practical aspects of sexual technique. Sex is spoken about more than ever before.

However, as Foucault (1979) has identified, in speaking we unwittingly define and proscribe who may have sex with whom, when and how. Indeed, as a society, our beliefs about what constitute 'normal' or 'appropriate' sexual behaviours (Weeks 1985) are firmly entrenched, determining not only popular portrayals of sex and sexuality in books and films, but also our research and policy interests.

The *National Survey of Sexual Attitudes and Lifestyles* was the most comprehensive sexual health survey ever to be carried out in the UK. Between 1990 and 1991, over 18,000 members of the British public were interviewed about their sexual attitudes and behaviours. Fundamental to the development of a national sexual health strategy, this research received widespread support both as a means of mapping out the likely spread of HIV infection, and as an unprecedented opportunity of obtaining a snapshot of the sexual 'lifestyles' of the UK population at the end of the twentieth century (Wellings et al. 1994).

The survey adopted an age cut-off of 59 years on the grounds that 'many of the topics for which data were collected are known not to affect older people greatly' (Johnson 1997: 23). For the follow-up study, instigated in 1998 to provide 'up to date information ... to underpin our decisions on policies that affect sexual health' (Metters 1998 http://news.bbc.co.uk/l/hi/health/203872.stm), the oldest of the 12,000 randomly selected participants was 44 (Johnson et al. 2001).

That this supposed 'comprehensive, national' survey excluded older people on the basis that sex and sexual health are not later life concerns both reflects, and reinforces, our tendency to desexualize old age. Indeed, although sex has become more visible in many areas of life, it is still considered to be the province of the young, slim and physically fit (Heath 1999). This notion is so deep-rooted within popular understandings of sexuality that it has been unequivocally accepted, even at a research and policy level. We *know* that sexual activity and interest decline significantly into later life. There is no need to collect data to prove this; it has become 'naturalized', a 'fact'.

Even within gerontology, the sexuality of older people is rarely acknowledged. Asking older people about sex is still seen as too difficult, too intrusive, and, fundamentally, unnecessary. The little work that has been done typically conforms to the tradition of sexologists such as Kinsey, where researchers try to gain an understanding of sexuality by quantifying it in terms of specific sexual acts and their frequencies. Broader aspects of later life sexuality, 'as much about words, images, ritual and fantasy as it is about the body' (Weeks 1985: 3), remain unexamined.

Not only is little specific attention paid to later life sexuality and sexual health issues, but these are also rarely considered in broader evaluations of later life well-being. How many quality of life tools used with older people include a 'sexual health' domain? How often is 'impact on sexuality' included as an endpoint in clinical trials with older populations? How frequently do health professionals discuss with their older patients the impact newly diagnosed conditions or newly prescribed medications may have upon their sexual health? The message is clear, within research, within policy and within practice: sexuality and sexual health are not considered to be important in old age.

However, alongside this denial of later life sexuality has been the emergence of a body of writing which 'challenges' this 'myth of the asexual old age'. Such writing tends to stress the importance of sexuality to people of all ages, but then highlights that older people are denied opportunities to be sexual because of societal intolerance of later life sexuality. The negative effect this 'denial of civil rights' (Hodson and Skeen 1994: 231) can have on older people is then outlined and data presented to 'prove' that older people are sexual (or rather, have (hetero)sexual intercourse). A central component of writing in this vein has been the claim that 'lifelong sexual function is a primary component of achieving successful ageing in general' (Katz and Marshall 2003: 12), a belief that has been particularly promoted within the popular media.

It will be argued that such writing is deconstructing one stereotype about sexuality and ageing only to create another in its place. This new myth of the 'sexy oldie' identifies remaining sexual as not merely a choice, but a responsibility for older people. Moreover, achieving continued membership of the 'sexualized world' is defined in youth-orientated terms, adhering to (youthful) notions of sexual attractiveness and engaging in sexual intercourse. As such, it is not old age that is being sexualized, but rather an extended middle age. The incompatibility of sexuality and old age is hence reinforced and, crucially, there is no room for older people's definitions of, and beliefs, about sexuality.

This book is split into three parts. In Part I, the two dominant stereotypes that typify contemporary understandings of sexuality and ageing will be explored: the 'myth of the asexual old age' and the more recent stereotype of the 'sexy oldie'. Part II will identify what we actually know about ageing and sexuality by synthesizing available literature, as well as exploring findings from one of the first qualitative studies to explore sexuality and sexual health issues with older people themselves. Their stories will highlight the differences, as well as the similarities, in older people's perspectives on these issues. Indeed, there is a danger when talking of 'older people' to assume commonality by age, where none exists. Exploring the differences among and between older men and women will be a major focus of the book.

While the role of medicine in defining and regulating sexuality has come under increasing scrutiny in recent years, there is no doubt that the tendency to view sexuality through a biomedical lens is set to continue. As such, issues relating to sexuality and sexual health have come to assume practical interest and importance for health professionals working with older people. Current evidence suggests that the sexual health needs of older people may not be acknowledged, let alone met, within health care settings. The final section of the book will explore what 'sexual health' means within the context of ageing and will focus on issues relevant to health professionals working with older people. A study conducted with UK general practitioners and practice nurses will be drawn upon to illuminate the barriers to discussing sexual health concerns with older patients.

Finally, it is important to stress that this book departs from most other writing in the sexuality and ageing field. Discussions will not look to reconcile sexuality and old age by drawing on biological data to show that older people have the potential to be 'sexual', or draw upon findings from surveys of sexual behaviour to argue that many older people do remain sexually active and therefore must be 'sexual'. Nor will sexuality be seen as a life-long 'essence' of both individuality and collective humanity and, hence, sexuality as something inherent to anyone, whatever their age. Indeed, the book does not seek to 'prove' that older people are sexual or, indeed, advocate they should be. Rather, the intention is to open up this area for debate, while, where possible, affording centrality to older people's own attitudes and beliefs. Hopefully, in so doing, a case will be made for viewing sexuality as part of the totality of later life experience.

PART I

Exploring contemporary understandings of sexuality and ageing

1

Why are sexuality and old age incompatible?

Unpicking the myth of the 'asexual old age'

Introduction

The first chapters of this book will explore two representations of later life sexuality that dominate contemporary beliefs and understandings: the 'asexual old age' and the 'sexy oldie'. The first and still most pervasive of these stereotypes is predicated upon the perceived incompatibility of old age and sexuality. By unpicking the meaning of these concepts, their antithetical stance will become self-evident. On the one hand, we have sexuality, represented by the youthful, healthy, beautiful body. On the other we have ageing, or perhaps more specifically old age, invoking images of physical decline, decrepitude and sickness. These ideas are difficult to reconcile and in contemporary society this is rarely done, despite the increasing number of 'challenges' to the exclusion of old age from the sexualized world. In the next chapter, these challenges will themselves be critiqued. It will be argued that writing in this vein is creating a new myth of the 'sexy oldie' where remaining 'sexual' is presented not as a choice, but a responsibility. Moreover, so doing is defined in relation to youth-focused understandings of sexuality and, as such, is more likely to reinforce the perceived incompatibility of sexuality and old age than challenge it.

At first glance these discussions may appear to have little in common with the lived experiences of older people. However, theorizing later life sexuality is not merely an academic exercise. Critically examining taken-for-granted concepts and their historical development helps us to understand why later life sexuality is understood in certain ways at the present time. Contextualizing it as such is important. It not only allows naturalized ideas about sexuality and ageing to be challenged, but also opens up the possibility for alterative understandings to emerge. Moreover, while it is certainly not argued that representations of later life sexuality reflect the experiences of older people themselves, they certainly influence their perceptions and expectations. As Giddens (1992) has argued, social norms play an important role in defining our own sexual attitudes and behaviours. These theoretical considerations therefore provide an important backdrop to the next part of the book, which will focus on what we 'know' about older people's understandings and experiences of sexuality.

The aim of the current chapter is to explore the myth of the asexual old age, something that will be addressed through an in-depth consideration of the concepts of 'old age' and 'sexuality'. While both are typically understood to be fixed in nature, when their meanings are probed more deeply, this is quickly revealed to be far from the case. Indeed, it will be argued that it is their socially constructed meanings that determine their incompatibility. The asexual old age has not emerged as the dominant conceptualization of later life sexuality because we do not have enough proof that older people have sex, which is how this issue is typically discussed within the gerontological and wider social science literature. Rather, this understanding of sexuality and ageing has emerged because of the oppositional meanings attached to sexuality and old age within contemporary society.

Meanings of old age

While old age is accepted as a 'natural' stage of the life course and, as such, fixed and universal, critical gerontologists (Phillipson 1998) have increasingly acknowledged the role of social factors in determining how this life stage is currently understood. For example, authors such as Cole (1992: xxii) argue that, although ageing and old age 'are certainly real ... they do not exist in some natural realm independently of the ideals, images, and social practices that conceptualize and represent them'. Similarly, Katz (1996: 51) argues that 'to be part of a population of elderly persons requires that one be absorbed into a specific discourse of differentiation'. This obviously leads on to questions of how and why ageing and old age are currently understood in the ways they are and this has been explored in detail in a growing number of publications (Minkler and Estes 1991; Featherstone and Wernick 1995; Katz 1996; Phillipson 1998; Biggs 1999; Blaikie 1999; Gilleard and Higgs 2000). Key strands to this discussion relevant to the relationship between sexuality, ageing and old age will be summarized here.

First, of fundamental influence to contemporary understandings of ageing has been the predilection to view old age through the 'biomedical lens'. As Estes and Binney (1991: 118) state, this 'equation of old age with illness has encouraged society to think about aging as pathological or abnormal', as a set of medical 'problems' which affect older people and to which medicine holds the solutions. They go on to argue that among the most significant implications of this way of understanding old age has been its impact upon public opinion – it is now taken for granted that ageing is a negative, irreversible process of decline and decay.

Gerontology has helped foster this image by 'consistently report[ing] and emphasiz[ing] decline, whether physical, psychological, or social, in the characteristics and capacities of the aged' (Levin and Levin 1980: ix). This is apparent when visiting most ageing congresses; it is often difficult to find presentations which do not focus upon the pathologies of old age – the strokes, the falls, the dementias. It now seems to be taken for granted by academics, health and social care professionals and wider society that 'To be old is to be unhealthy' (Victor 1991: 2).

It is therefore unsurprising that images of old age are so inextricably linked with notions of dependency. Indeed, as Phillipson (1998) claims, the very definition of old age is itself predicated on financial dependency. He highlights that the idea of 'the old' constituting a separate group within society only emerged at the beginning of the twentieth century, with the introduction of the old age pension in the UK and USA, distributed according to standard chronological retirement ages. Therefore, old age was, and continues to be, defined by marginalization and dependency: marginalization from employment and productivity, and dependency upon the state. This is well exemplified in contemporary debates about the ageing population, where the spectre of younger people 'carrying the burden' of a large, sick and demanding old population looms large.

Crucially, representing old age as a time of dependency contributes to the idea that this is a stage of life where adulthood is in doubt. As Featherstone and Hepworth (1990) state, the loss of bodily control associated with ageing, and more importantly, inextricably linked to images of old age, impairs the capacity to be treated as a competent adult. The idea that older people can revert to a 'second childhood', due to loss of physical and, perhaps crucially, cognitive function is not only evident in the verbal and visual imagery of old age, but can also lead to older people being treated as children and, ultimately, denied personhood (Hockey and James 1993). For example, older people are often referred to by their Christian names by health care professionals in a way that mirrors the approach they would use with children, reflecting the tendency to view older people not as proper 'adults'. Moreover, there is an assumption within contemporary society that 'to be fully human, one must be able to function fully' (Charmaz 1983: 187), the implication being that the physical frailty that accompanies ageing for some (but not all) older people calls the essential humanity of *all* older people into doubt.

Furthermore, not only has the meagreness of the state pension ensured that, for many, old age is characterized by economic dependency or, in blunter terms extreme poverty, but statutory retirement has also disempowered older people in more covert ways. As Bytheway acknowledges: 'Participation in the labour market still remains a major determinant of status and identity in modern societies. Paid employment grants us activity, mobility, experience and expertise, as well as income' (1995: 52). In other words, and as argued for a number of years by key 'critical gerontologists' (Townsend 1981; Walker 1986; Estes 1991; Phillipson 1998), structural politico-economic factors considered specific to capitalist societies have combined to create a dominant experience of old age characterized by political, social and economic disenfranchisement.

Another means by which old age has become excluded and invisible within mainstream society is through the pathologization of the old body. As Öberg (1996) has identified, old bodies are known to us only through the medicalized body and the malfunctioning body – there are no positive images of older people's bodies and those images of older bodies which are not medically framed can be shocking. Indeed, our attitudes towards old bodies have advanced little since one of the first textbooks of Geriatric Medicine, published in 1914, listed the following 'decaying' characteristics of the old body: 'thin hair, brittle nails, dry and loose skin, uneven muscle texture, slackened jaw, loss of teeth, and slouching posture' (Katz 1996: 85).

The old body profoundly influences how we feel about both old age and older people. Gubrium (1986) goes so far as to argue that these perceived physical changes with ageing result in older people (or perhaps more specifically people who appear to be old) being characterized as a separate species. Moreover, in contemporary society, signs of ageing have symbolic meaning above and beyond their visible signs upon the body; rather they are increasingly recognized as markers of individual failure to maintain the body to a youthful ideal. Wrinkling skin, grey hair and weight gain are among the myriad of physical changes accompanying ageing that, women in particular, dread because, as Dinnerstein and Weitz (1998: 189) acknowledge, the ageing body 'challenges acceptable notions of femininity'. Indeed, for both men and women, the old body is the antithesis of the beautiful body, characterized as slim, healthy, unwrinkled and, most crucially, young.

Ageing, but resisting 'old age'

Given these associations with sickness, dependency, ugliness and failure, it is unsurprising that old age represents a lifestage with which few people would choose to engage, whatever their age (Gilleard and Higgs 2000). Indeed, there is an increasing recognition that while old age may remain fixed in the popular imagination as something to be feared and reviled, ageing itself cannot be understood in the ways it has for most of recorded history, namely as a 'common or totalizing experience' which all people experience in a homogenous way (2000: 1). Rather, it has been argued that people are increasingly choosing the ways in which they age, notably through the ways in which they consume (Hepworth 1996; Katz 1996; Biggs 1999; Gilleard and Higgs 2000). This may at first sound nonsensical – people cannot choose not to age. However, consider the phenomenal commercial success of anti-ageing products – the creams, pills and potions people of all ages are increasingly sold as a means of staving off the dreaded prospect of being recognized as someone who is 'old'. Increasingly, people do not want to be age-classified according to the clothes they wear, the music they listen to, or the food they eat. Moreover, joining this race to resist ageing is increasingly sold by society not only as a choice, but a responsibility. In the same way that maintaining your own health has been deemed a personal responsibility and sickness a personal failure (Ogden 2000), so we are increasingly cajoled to take responsibility for our own ageing. If you do not have the money, time, or inclination to maintain the façade of youth, then the transition to old age seems inevitable and you have failed.

It is for these reasons that the title of this book refers to sexuality and ageing, rather than sexuality and old age. Ageing offers the potential to be sexual, whereas old age does not. Not only are images of old age profoundly anti-sexual but, as explored below, meanings of sexuality within contemporary society leave no room for old age. That is not to say that I am proposing that older people cannot be sexual (although whether they are as desperate to identify with societal definitions of what this means is another question). However, conforming to what 'being sexual' represents within our society can only be achieved through resisting the transition to old age.

The remainder of this chapter will explore what we mean by 'sexuality', proposing that although, like 'old age', it may be commonly understood as rooted in biology and therefore 'natural', when this idea is unpicked, it is exposed as highly tenuous. This is certainly not to propose that biology is irrelevant – the ageing body brings the limits of social constructionism sharply into focus. However, it is to acknowledge that there is nothing inherently 'sexual' or 'asexual' about old age; later life is excluded from our contemporary sexualized world because the meanings which underpin dominant representation of old age are anti-sexual, while those underpinning sexuality itself are inextricably linked to youth.

What is sexuality?

It is unsurprising that we invest heavily in trying to pin sexuality down given that now more than ever sexuality has come to represent the truth of our being (Foucault 1979). At an individual level we seem desperate to get to grips with our sexuality and a large and lucrative industry of 'experts' has grown up to help us achieve this. At a collective level, sexologists, the 'scientists of sex', have tried to illuminate our universal sexuality by breaking it down into constituent attitudes and behaviours which can be quantified. Whatever way you look at it, understanding sexuality is big business.

It seems ironic, then, that we are further than ever from understanding what 'sexuality' actually is. As a society, despite desperate attempts and even increasing technologies which 'expand your capacity to have a view on your sexuality' (Roddick 2002: 2), sexuality still seems to elude us. Even when sexuality becomes the subject of academic research, the topic under investigation is rarely explicitly defined. Laumann et al. (1994), for example, in their book *The Social Organization of Sexuality*, based on interviews with 3432 Americans, at no point state what this 'sexuality' they are so keen to investigate actually is (although their sample age cut-off implies that it is something that has no relevance to anyone over 60). However, they imply that it is something that can be broken down and measured. They infer that it exists as a concrete phenomenon. Something you can understand, something you can 'have'.

This belief is highly visible in attempts to define sexuality in relation to older people and many authors try very hard to deliver the definitive definition. However, these definitions often leave the reader as confused as to what sexuality is not, as enlightened about what it actually is. For example, Hogan (1980: 3) argues that sexuality comprises 'Much more than the sex act ... the quality of being human, all that we are as men and women ... encompassing the most intimate feelings and deepest longings of the heart to find meaningful relationships'; in other words, just about anything. Hillman (2000) tries to clarify the matter further by identifying those *specific* behaviours and emotions that constitute 'sexuality':

> Sexuality will be defined here as a *broadly based* term that indicates any combination of sexual behaviour, sensual activity, emotional intimacy, or sense of sexual identity. Any individual's wish to engage in any of these activities also may be considered an aspect of sexuality. Sexuality may involve sexual activity with the explicit goal of achieving pleasure or climax (e.g. kissing, foreplay, intercourse), sensual activity with or without the explicit goal of achieving sexual pleasure (e.g. wearing body lotion to feel attractive or feminine), or the experience of emotional intimacy within the context of a romantic relationship. Thus sexuality incorporates a vast number of issues including body image, masturbation, love, libido, intercourse, homophobia, relationship satisfaction, marital satisfaction, desires for sexual and sensual experience, and participation in high-risk behaviours.
>
> (2000: 5–6; emphasis added)

Again, this attempt to pin down sexuality highlights the difficulties inherent in so doing – where do you stop? It is therefore perhaps unsurprising that, when push comes to shove and sexuality has to be 'operationalized' within empirical research studies, this complexity quickly becomes forgotten. Indeed, when faced with this worrying lack of clarity, most authors quickly state, either implicitly or explicitly, that their definition of sexuality focuses on *sexual activity*, or rather, (hetero) sexual intercourse. This is evident throughout writings about sexuality and ageing and one example will suffice. Bancroft (1983: 282), having identified ageing as one of the 'problems' of human sexuality, argues that 'there is an undoubted decline in the sexuality of both men and women with advancing years'. He goes on to cite rates of sexual intercourse as markers of 'sexuality'.

How sexuality is understood in this book

The premise of this book is quite different. It will be argued that this notion of one 'true' sexuality is highly tenuous; that, as Tiefer eloquently puts it, 'sex is not a natural act' (1995: 1). Rather, sexuality can better be understood as a social construction 'which brings together a host of different biological and mental possibilities – gender identity, bodily differences, reproductive capacities, needs, desires and fantasies – which need not be linked together, and in other cultures have not been' (Weeks 1986: 15). This may at first seem absurd given how ingrained beliefs about sexuality are within popular culture. However, studies of the 'history' of sexuality have identified that the concept of sexuality itself is relatively modern. Foucault, for example, writes that the 'term itself did not appear until the beginning of the nineteenth century, a fact that should neither be overestimated or overinterpreted' (1984: 3). This obviously does not mean that the behaviours and experiences to which sexuality refers did not exist before this time, but rather that they had not been conceptualized in this way before.

Insights such as these help answer a number of questions about sexuality that cannot be satisfactorily answered from a traditional standpoint. Tiefer, for example, poses the following questions of sexuality:

> What is to be included? How much of the body is relevant? How much of the life span? Is sexuality an individual dimension or a dimension of a relationship? Which behaviors, thoughts and feelings qualify as sexual – an unreturned glance? any hug? daydreams about celebrities? fearful memories of abuse? When can we use the same language for animals and people, if at all?
>
> (1995: 20)

In addition, there are those further issues around sexuality as an identity – heterosexual/straight, homosexual/gay and so on, as well as the complex relationship between sexuality and gender. How can one definition of sexuality incorporate all these attitudes, behaviours and ideas? The answer is, obviously, that it cannot because sexuality itself is not a simple, singular, measurable phenomenon.

Adopting this approach leads us to the conclusion that nothing is inherently 'sexual', but naming it makes it so (Plummer 1975). This obviously has significant implications for the labelling of old age as 'asexual'. It infers this label of 'asexual' has little to do with whether older people are 'sexually active' or not, which is how this issue seems to be currently interpreted. Rather, it is likely to relate to wider ideas about what it is that makes something, or someone, 'sexual'. As the feminist authors Travis, Meginis and Bardari state:

> The social framework of sexuality provides rules about who can be sexual and under what circumstances sexual behaviour is appropriate. The social framework of sexuality even defines what counts as sex. Ultimately, individual experiences of being sexual and sexually aroused are determined, at least in part, by these socially constructed realities.
>
> (2000. 238–9)

The first two chapters of this book examine the 'social framework' and consider where it positions ageing and old age.

This discussion may be disappointing in some respects. I would argue that there is no simple, singular definition that can be applied to sexuality. We can only summarize what sexuality is not, not what it is. We can say that sexuality is not fixed in biology, universal or shared. Nor is it simple, clear-cut and 'measurable'. Sexuality is neither apolitical nor atheoretical. Sexuality is not something you possess or a unique essence of personality. Sexuality does not have one discrete meaning. Rather, it is more appropriate to talk of multiple 'sexualities', an idea which opens up the possibility that 'sexuality' can be 'thought about, experienced, and acted upon differently' according to gender, 'class, ethnicity, physical ability, sexual orientation and preference, religion, ... region' (Vance 1989: 17) and, crucially, age.

Contemporary understandings of sexuality: implications for ageing and old age

Adopting the position that understandings of sexuality reflect societal judgements rather than any objective or naturally occurring 'facts' leads us to explore both the meanings attributed to sexuality, and the processes shaping these meanings. This is obviously not a straightforward process and whole books have been devoted to such an analysis (Parker and Gagnon 1995; Tiefer 1995; Hawkes 1996; Bristow 1997), particularly in writings exploring the history (or perhaps more accurately 'histories') of sexuality (Foucault 1979; 1984; 1986; Weeks 1985; 1986; Nye 1999). However, this body of work has paid scant attention to age and, certainly, to old age, despite saying much of relevance to how sexuality and ageing are understood within contemporary society.

This section will discuss key beliefs underpinning contemporary meanings of sexuality, including: (1) notions of sexuality as a natural and powerful urge; (2) beliefs that there are 'normal' and 'abnormal' sexualities; (3) a view of sexuality as an inherent personality characteristic which underpins maturity and mental health; (4) an emphasis on sexual intercourse as the 'gold standard' of sexuality; (5) perceiving the body as an external marker of inherent sexuality; and (6) the growing medicalization of sexuality.

Sexology and the 'naturalness' of (potentially reproductive) sexuality

Sexuality is typically conceptualized as something universal, fixed and biologically determined. An assumption deeply rooted within our culture is that our sexuality is the most spontaneously natural thing about us (Weeks 1985). This is reflected in the language used to describe sexuality, a language of 'drives', 'forces' and 'urges'. Our supposedly natural 'sexual instincts' are regarded as universal, shared by all humans, and even some animals. As Tiefer has stated: 'It's all sexuality, after all, in one big happy mammalian family' (1995: 34).

However, these supposedly natural instincts have been regarded with suspicion for centuries. As Weeks (1985: 8) notes: 'The belief that sex is an overpowering force which the social/moral/medical has to control is an old and deeply rooted one, and central to the western, Christian traditions.' This is a task that religion, and latterly 'science', notably in the guise of sexology, have been eager to take on. These regulatory forces have set norms for sexual attitudes and behaviours and, in particular, defined sexual intercourse with the potential to result in procreation as the crux of 'healthy' sexuality. As such, a disapproval of sexual pleasure in its own right has dominated Western thinking about sexuality for centuries (Foucault 1979).

The early sexologists began to transform non-reproductive sex from something to be disapproved of as morally suspect, to something to be viewed as a disease or disorder. From the late nineteenth century onwards they began to set strict criteria for appropriate sexualities. Abnormal manifestations of sexuality, as judged against what was perceived as natural, became pathologized as 'perversions' and their perpetrators as 'perverts'. This is evident in Richard Krafft-Ebing's key text *Psychopathia Sexualis* (1886). For example, he writes that: 'During the time of the [maturation of the] physiological processes in the reproductive glands, desires arise in the consciousness of the individual which have for their purpose the perpetuation of the species (sexual instinct)' (1886: 23). Later on he notes that: 'With opportunity for the natural satisfaction of sexual instinct, every expression of it that does not correspond with the purpose of nature – i.e. propagation – must be regarded as perverse' (1886: 56).

While sexology has actually paid little attention to sexuality in old age, an ideology such as this obviously creates a backdrop against which sexuality in later life, which is very rarely for reproductive ends, is deemed a perversion. Moreover, this belief was actively perpetuated in the little written by the early sexologists on sexuality within the context of old age. For example, Havelock Ellis in the *Psychology of Sex* (1933) includes a special section on 'sexual senility' in his chapter entitled 'Sexual deviations'. Unsurprisingly, this negatively frames expressions of sexuality among both post-menopausal women, and older men. He writes, for instance, that 'in men, when the approach of age begins to be felt, the sexual impulse may suddenly become urgent. In this instinctive reaction it may tend to roam, normally or abnormally, beyond legitimate bounds' (Ellis 1933: 181). Later on he identifies that this 'late exacerbation of sexuality becomes still more dangerous if it takes the form of an attraction to girls who are no more than children' (1933: 181).

While Havelock Ellis is less vocal about older women, what he does say is similarly negative. For example, he writes that: 'There is a frequent well marked tendency in women at the menopause to an eruption of sexual desire, the last flaring up of a dying fire, which may easily take on a morbid form' (1933: 181). These ideas have been perpetuated within the popular scientific literature as late as 1970, when the American doctor David Reuben wrote that:

> Without oestrogen, the quality of being female gradually disappears...[and] a woman becomes as close as she can to being a man. ... decline of breasts and female genitalia all contribute to a masculine appearance ... Having outlived their ovaries, they may have outlived their usefulness as human beings.
>
> (1970: 288–9)

Even within contemporary society, despite the uncoupling of reproduction from sex through 'test tube babies, surrogate mothers, and cloning' (Longstaff Mackay 2001: 623), it is apparent that judgements about normal and abnormal sexuality continue to be made against the reproductive norm fixed within Western Christian tradition and cemented by the writings of the early sexologists. Indeed, contemporary sexual attitudes and behaviours still afford primacy and, critically, legitimacy to those sexual behaviours which at least have the potential to result in reproduction – namely heterosexual intercourse (Tiefer 2000) between younger people. The justification for this thinking takes us back to nature again – potentially reproductive sexual behaviours are viewed as 'natural', the touchstone for 'normality' and general societal approval.

The importance of an intrinsic sexuality to maturity and mental health
The writing of the early sexologists popularized the idea that sexuality is not only something you 'do', but also something you 'have'. This idea was particularly expounded by Freud (1977) in his essays on sexuality and, again, continues to underpin contemporary thought, notably within psychology. For example, Stuart and Sundeen (1979) argue that 'To a large extent, human sexuality determines who we are. It is an integral factor in the uniqueness of every person' (cited Kessel 2001: 121). These ideas are particularly apparent within writings about sexuality and ageing and, in particular, used as an argument as to why it is important for 'professionals' to pay attention to the sexuality *in* older people. As Sherman argues, 'sexuality and making love are part of the fabric of our lives; part of the very essence of being human – *even for* older people' (1998: 4, italics added). The logical extension of this argument for some has been that to be a 'living being' (not even a human being), it is necessary, not only to recognize your inherent sexuality, but to actively express it, whatever your age. MacNab, for example, argues that: 'Both sexes as they reach their elderly years rarely use sexual interest as a factor in their appearance and behaviour, without any conscious awareness that what they are thereby doing is denying or repressing a large part of what it is to be a living being' (1994: 141). The role of writings like this in creating new myths about sexuality and ageing will be explored in the next chapter.

This inherent sexuality, which we are all said to 'have,' is considered an important component of maturity and mental health (Tiefer 2000). Again, this belief can be traced back to the conceptual shift brought about by the early sexologists in terms of labelling someone who expressed abnormal or 'perverted' sexual behaviours as a 'pervert'. Prior to this it was the behaviours that were deemed 'abnormal', not the individual. As Weeks (1985) identifies, the most obvious example of this shift could be seen in relation to attitudes towards (male) homosexuality. While before the late nineteenth century 'practising sodomy did not, in any ontological sense, make you a different sort of being' (1985: 90), after this date, 'the homosexual emerged as a distinct type of person', a person defined by their sexual behaviours. That these behaviours became defined as a manifestation of individual mental health is indicated by the classification of homosexuality as a 'mental disorder' by the American Psychiatric Association until 1973.

Viewing sexuality as an important marker of psychological maturity and, crucially, of adult psychological maturity, has obvious implications for attitudes towards sexuality and ageing. As identified previously in this chapter, the belief that ageing constitutes a process of inevitable physical and mental decline has led to old age being characterized as a 'second childhood'. However, as we all know, 'sexuality' and 'childhood' do not fit easily alongside each other. Indeed, ultimately sex is defined as an adult activity and certainly not something that is relevant to those whose mental maturity is in doubt, whether this is because they are too young, or too old.

Sexuality equals sexual intercourse

Sexual intercourse is now more than ever the 'gold standard' for sexuality. Hawkes identifies through an analysis of articles about sex in women's magazines in the 1990s, that coital sex is regarded as 'the summit of sexual experience' (1996: 121). Teenage girls are exhorted to 'please their man' through finding the most satisfying sexual 'position' for intercourse – *More* magazine helpfully illustrates a new 'position' every fortnight for such educational purposes. Bill Clinton's belief that the term 'sexual relations' encompasses only sexual intercourse (and crucially not oral sex) served to reflect, and reinforce, popular beliefs that intercourse is the only 'true' expression of sexuality. As Gavey et al. (1999: 60) state, 'the possibility that intercourse could be a choice for sexually active heterosexuals is rarely publicly aired'.

Hawkes (1996) argues that the primacy afforded to heterosexual intercourse reflects a masculinist bias, given known differences between men and women in pleasure derived from sexual intercourse. It could be argued that it also reflects an ageist bias. Numerous (mainly US) surveys have identified that rates of sexual intercourse decline after middle age. For example, it has been estimated that by the age of 70, 67 per cent of men will experience some degree of erectile dysfunction (Feldman et al. 1994). Moreover, a recent study identified that 28 per cent of women aged 18–75 experience vaginal dryness and that this increases in prevalence with age (Dunn et al. 1998). High degrees of individual difference are ignored and, as such old age becomes characterized as a time when sexual intercourse occurs less frequently, if at all. This obviously renders older people 'asexual', given that sexual intercourse is a key marker of 'sexuality' within contemporary society.

Many of the writings about sexuality and ageing implicitly take on board this message that sexual intercourse is the 'best' sex, through considerations of how older people can 'compensate' for a potentially reduced ability to have intercourse in light of erectile dysfunction, vaginal dryness or other health problems. Hendricks and Hendricks, for example, despite beginning to argue that intercourse should not be seen as the only form of sexual expression, betray their belief that it is the most satisfying, or perhaps only, form of sex in the final sentence: 'At all ages coitus is but a single element in the communication of love ... For elderly couples being physically or spiritually close, showing tenderness or respect can be valued in such a way that intercourse is hardly missed' (1978: 71).

The crucial importance afforded to sexual intercourse as the only 'true' sex is also apparent in academic writings about sexuality; the vast majority of research focuses upon identifying rates of intercourse – other forms of sexuality are often ignored, undoubtedly in part because they are so difficult to pin down.

Exterior 'sexiness' as the marker for inherent sexuality

Another key belief about sexuality is that this supposedly inherent characteristic can be represented externally, not only through behaviour, but also through appearance. Indeed, external 'sexiness' is increasingly seen as a marker of 'interior' sexuality, reflecting a general trend over recent decades for our bodies to assume unprecedented social significance. As Featherstone

(1991) argues, inner personality or 'self' has become ever more conflated with the external body.

It is therefore a glaring omission that, within research and writing about sexuality, 'the body' has tended to be ignored. This is particularly true in writings about sexuality and ageing, where the focus has been upon specific sexual acts and behaviours. As these writings are often attempting to challenge the myth of later life asexuality they fail to acknowledge that, increasingly, it is having a body which conforms to an ideal of sexual attractiveness that identifies you as possessing sexuality and, as such, being 'sexual', rather than any sexual behaviours you engage in. This is particularly true for women.

Indeed, it is feminist authors who have argued that, 'sexuality [has been moved] into the public realm, making it concrete and external, and thereby amenable to inspection, definition, social monitoring, and control' (Travis et al. 2000: 239). As such, the extent to which women can conform to this ideal becomes a marker of their sexuality – 'the shape of a woman's body, the size of her breasts, and the color of her hair, are all features commonly used to assess her value as a sexual being' (2000: 239). Moreover:

> To be sexual, for women, means to be an object of desire. Thus, whether or not one is sexual is determined almost exclusively by the judgements and experiences of others ... Sexuality is construed in the flair of the nostril, the arch of the brow, the proportions of the waist and hips, the tone of the skin, ad infinitum. This formulation renders older women; larger, heavy women; and handicapped women asexual.
>
> (Travis et al. 2000: 240)

This indicates that older women's perceptions of themselves as sexual may be largely dependent on the beliefs of others.

The norms against which women's sexual attractiveness and, thereby, inherent sexuality are measured, leave little room for the old body. With every wrinkle, grey hair and pound gained, women move away from the 'sexy' body and, crucially, become perceived as less sexual. It has been argued that things are different for men, that women of all ages are still judged by their appearance in ways that men escape (Sontag 1978). Indeed, while there are increasing cultural messages coercing men also to assume responsibility for maintaining their body to a youthful ideal, there is still an acceptance that men who do not conform to the 'Adonis' ideal can be sexually attractive – larger men, shorter men, even older men. Increasing age for men has typically also meant increasing economic wealth and power and economically powerful men are deemed sexy within contemporary society, whether they meet standards for male physical perfection or not. Ultimately, however, there remains a point where the old body, whether male or female, cannot be viewed as sexy and, by extension, the older person as sexual. Deep old age is never sexy. The 'decaying' characteristics of the old body (Katz 1996) take you as far away as you can get from the body beautiful.

The medicalization of sexuality

Finally, it is important to recognize a trend that is increasingly underpinning how sexuality is understood, discussed and experienced, namely, medicalization. Indeed, while medicine has historically played an important role in shaping and even defining what we mean by sexuality (Weeks 1989), in recent years, medicine's interest in this area has extended so that sexual desire and performance are now deemed serious public health concerns (Laumann et al. 1999). One result of this has been that until:

> Relatively recently, the imperative was for restraint and moderation in sexual matters; now it is for more and better sexual gratification. We can see this as the replacement of one orthodoxy by another – as an over-medicalisation of sex. Celibacy is the new deviance.
>
> (Hart and Wellings 2002: 899)

Medicalization has helped create an ethos within contemporary society where to be happy and healthy, you need to be having (good) sex. Since the 1960s, the belief that heterosexual intercourse and orgasms are good for you has dominated thinking about sexuality (Reich 1982), despite coming under extensive criticism; numerous authors have exposed the historically contingent and socially constructed nature of these discourses. Nicolson and Burr, for example, trace the origins of the sex–health connection back to the work of sexologists such as Krafft-Ebing, Havelock-Ellis and Freud, and identify that, although pervading contemporary medical and lay understandings of 'normal' sexuality, they have little empirical base. For example, they identify that although sexual fulfilment *through orgasm* has long been thought to be good for women and underpins contemporary classifications of sexual 'dysfunction', available research evidence indicates that orgasm through intercourse, 'the "classic" form of orgasmic experience' (2003: 1737) is not necessarily common among women (Kinsey et al. 1953; Nicolson 1993; 1994), or even fundamental to women's definitions of pleasurable sex (Keodt 1974; Hite 1989; Nicolson and Burr 2003).

However, this critique has not fed into dominant understandings of sexuality and, indeed, having sex is *increasingly* seen as a prerequisite for being happy and healthy within contemporary society. This is evident in any cursory look at the popular media. For example, a recent article in the online woman's magazine 'handbag.com' (Richards 2003 http://www.handbag.com/relationships/sex/sexisgood) lists the numerous 'health benefits' of sex, concluding that: 'great sex does so much good that you should consider making love as often as possible. So what are you waiting for? Go grab your man!' (grabbing your woman is not given as an option).

In the medical and nursing literature, from which much of the research and discussion about sexuality emanates, the health benefits of sex are often presented as a rationale for why medicine and allied health professions should be interested in this area. It can be argued that one reason for this is that the connection between sex and health makes respectable a topic which is often perceived as morally dubious. If sex is healthy, then it becomes more acceptable to research and write about. After all, people of all ages value health above anything else (Gilleard and Higgs 2000) and are endlessly fascinated by sex. Given this background, it is unsurprising that research findings are increasingly presented in such a way as to promote sex, particularly for older people, as healthy. A recent press release by the Director of the Sexual Medicine Programme at New York's Cornell Medical Center, for example, states:

> Sex is good for you, with benefits including a longer, healthier, and happier life ... Conversely sexual problems like erectile dysfunction (ED) can contribute to a variety of other mental and physical problems, including depression and relationship discord. ED may also be a harbinger of diseases, including diabetes, multiple sclerosis, Parkinson's disease, [and] coronary artery disease, among others.

It goes on to claim that 'More people are having sex than ever before – and later in life. As the population ages, and treatments for sexual function improve, men and women will continue to enjoy sex late in life' (http://www.med.cornell.edu/news/press/2003/10_14_03_b.html).

Sexuality and old age: oppositional and irreconcilable?

This chapter has sought conceptual clarity, specifically in terms of elucidating what is meant both by 'sexuality' and by 'old age'. When these ideas are juxtaposed, the reasons why old age is characterized as asexual, or even anti-sexual, become obvious. The highly negative images we have of old age hold no place within our contemporary sexualized world. This section reiterates why this is so.

First, it has been identified that the link between 'normal' sexuality and reproduction marginalizes the vast majority of older people for whom this is not an aspect of sexual activity. Indeed, while the era of effective contraception and test tube babies may make us feel that sex now has little to do with conception, judgements about normal sexualities are still made against a reproductive norm.

Furthermore, sex is closely linked with notions of mental maturity and, in particular, is delineated as an 'adult' activity. However, in old age, adulthood can be in doubt, particularly in the face of physical and psychological dependency. Therefore, it is apparent that the desexualization of older people both reflects, and contributes towards, the infantilization of old age. The tendency to view older people as having reverted back to childhood confirms the incongruity between sexuality and old age; presenting old age as asexual reinforces the assumption that older people are not 'adults'. Moreover, sex is not only seen as a means to maintain health, but as an activity of the healthy. The characterization of older people as sick and dependent therefore also further disbars them from the sexualized world.

In addition, it has been argued that whether a person is considered 'sexual' or not depends to a large degree upon their physical appearance. In contemporary society, youth is the defining feature of the 'sexy body' and the old body is viewed as profoundly anti-sexual. Moreover, sexuality, and in particular the exterior manifestation of sexuality, namely, sexual attractiveness, have 'emerged as a guarantee for attaining status and security' (Weeks 1985: 27).

Characterizing old age as asexual therefore both reinforces, and reflects, the overall position of older people within contemporary society. Indeed, Gibson takes this argument a step further. He proposes that the rendering of old age as asexual reflects a more general desire by younger people to disempower the older generation and that 'some of the younger generations would like to regard "the old" as being asexual and impotent in every sense, and fit only to drag out the remainder of their years on a wretched pension, divorced from the real concerns of life until they thankfully drop dead' (1992: 11–12).

Although it can be argued that the power dynamics which render youth sexual and powerful and old age asexual and powerless are not as overt as he would imply, his identification that perceptions of sexuality in old age are indicative of older people's overall status within society is certainly important. As Travis et al. (2000: 239) state:

> Socially constructed definitions of sexuality do not occur randomly but derive from the interests of privileged groups. Those who are in power (political, economic, and social) have the most influence in establishing the social framework and are in positions to exert more influence over its design, usually for their own comfort.

Within this context, later life stereotyping around sexuality could be seen to derive, in part, from younger people's definitions of old age as 'the other' – they are sexually virile and attractive because they are not 'old'.

Finally, a key issue for men in particular, but for women also, given that the female experience of sexuality is typically framed in terms of heterosexuality, relates to the privileging of biology and, in particular, sexual intercourse as a marker of 'true' sexuality. If having sexual intercourse is one of the key factors in determining whether you are perceived as 'sexual' or not, then evidence that rates of sexual intercourse decline into later life obviously contribute to the characterization of old age as asexual.

Conclusion

It can be argued that old age is characterized as asexual because of our obsession with the sexual, and our deep fear of old age. Fundamentally, it reflects the widespread and ingrained ageism within society, representing just one of many strategies used to disenfranchise old age and disempower older people. Ultimately, old age is characterized as asexual because of a widespread perception that sexuality represents all that is perceived as 'good' within society, namely power, wealth, beauty, and, crucially, youth. Old age, by contrast represents all that is feared about being human – dependency on others, economic disenfranchisement, ugliness, sickness and death.

Despite challenges to the ageism within society that result in older people being characterized in such a negative light, these images continue to hold currency, even within the context of an increasingly older population. Maybe this is not as contradictory as would first appear. Indeed, paradoxically, as life expectancy has increased, ageing (or more specifically the embodiment of ageing), has become feared more than ever. Such fears have been promoted and fuelled by a consumer culture where the potential of the grey pound is increasingly apparent (Gilleard and Higgs 2000) – resisting old age in any way possible is not only encouraged, but expected. It seems that the ethos of successful ageing has become so powerful that anyone who fails to succeed, by having the misfortune to be diagnosed with an age-related chronic condition, or through their inability or unwillingness to maintain the body to a youthful ideal, is characterized as failing, full stop.

Therefore, it becomes more and more apparent why traditional approaches to 'challenging' the stereotype of later life asexuality will never achieve their goal of sexualizing old age. These have typically involved 'proving' that older people are sexually active, or arguing from a human rights perspective that sexuality is inherent to humanity and hence people of all ages. However, as is the case with many forms of stereotyping, characterizing old age as asexual has little to do with the people themselves who are defined in this way. Indeed, what this stereotyping means to older people themselves has received scant attention – in the next chapter it will be argued that liberation from being 'sexual' may be just that – liberating. Nevertheless, it is unlikely that this argument will ever gain widespread currency within society, given the economic vested interests in promoting age-resisting technologies to 'banish' old age, whether this is through cosmetic means or prescription drugs. That this has created a new and equally oppressive stereotype of the 'sexy oldie' cast within the mould of positive ageing, will be argued in the next chapter.

2

The 'sexy oldie'

The creation of new myths about sexuality and ageing

Introduction

The asexual old age is only one context, although arguably the dominant context, within which sexuality and ageing are understood. Indeed, since the 1970s, the little that has been written in the gerontological and health literature about later life sexuality and sexual health has actively promoted older people's sexual expression, albeit in a very narrow context. More recently, there has been a 'cultural-scientific' shift, particularly reflected in the popular media, whereby 'lifelong sexual function ... [has come to be seen as] a primary component of achieving successful ageing in general' (Katz and Marshall 2003: 12). As Katz and Marshall note, this shift in thinking has been underpinned both by an increasingly consumerist culture and the positive ageing movement. In addition, it can also be argued that the medical community and pharmaceutical company agendas have also played their part, particularly in terms of defining the right to sexual fulfilment as a public health concern (Laumann et al. 1999) for people of all ages.

The increasing drive to sexualize later life has been almost unquestioningly viewed as 'a good thing'. Indeed, particularly within the gerontological and health literature, so doing has been viewed as 'liberating' older people from the myth of the asexual old age. The scene is normally set by stating how vitally important sexuality is to people of all ages, but then arguing that older people are denied opportunities to be sexual because of societal intolerance of later life sexuality. The denial of these opportunities is framed as a human rights abuse. For example, Hodson and Skeen (1994: 231) argue that 'deny[ing] ... sexual potential is as surely a denial of civil rights as denying someone equal employment or housing opportunity'. The role for research in this area has therefore been deemed to be to 'confront' and 'replace' 'myths and stereotypes ... with accurate information' which can be provided to older people by 'health professionals who have the relevant knowledge and skills' (Ford 1998: 145).

Similarly, the increasing 'acceptance' of older people's sexuality within the media has been seen as empowering and life-affirming. For example, a recent opinion column published in *The Sunday Times* claims that: 'Old people are practically the only ones left having guilt-free, strings-free recreational sex. They're not only the new teenagers, but also the new rabbits.' It goes on to state that 'I realise I'm making it sound like it's all about sex, but really it's all about having fun and living life' (Knight 2003: 4). Older female celebrities seem to be in the vanguard of promoting a new sexualized role model for older women. Jilly Cooper (1997), for example, stated in the Summer issue of *World of Retirement* that 'Sexagenarian ... comes after sex in the dictionary' (cited in Blaikie 1999: 101). Others, like Jane Fonda and Nancy Friday, 'exhort mid-life women to use their new-found power to continue the potentially "ageless" pursuit of a sexualized lifestyle that incorporates both intimacy and attractiveness' (Gilleard and Higgs 2000: 74).

However, you are left to ponder whether older people want to be the 'new teenagers', having casual sex, 'for fun'. Do you have to be having sex to be 'living life'? Is denial of sexual rights really a human rights abuse? Moreover, despite the increasingly positive messages transmitted that older people (and particularly older women) can be seen as sexy and that '60 is the new 30', is this more rhetoric than reality? As noted by a recent columnist writing in *The Guardian*, older female celebrities

> look young, they dress like their 25-year-old counterparts, they apparently have sex – so what's the difference? Well, it's the cultural assumption that 35 years is quite long enough for any woman to be an object of desire, and with mileage mounting on the clock, it's best to strip them of sexiness before it gets gross.
>
> (Sullivan 2003
> http://www.guardian.co.uk/comment/story/0,3604.10881890,00.html)

If the sell-by date on appearing sexy is 35, then where does this leave people in their forties, fifties, sixties? They can struggle to maintain the 25-year-old ideal of sexual attractiveness, but the message is that they are unlikely to succeed. Those in their seventies, eighties and nineties will never succeed.

So, when viewed critically, how positive are these messages about sexuality and ageing? Do they really liberate older people from the myth of the 'asexual old age' and give them permission to join the 'sexualized world' enjoyed by younger people? Is membership of this world really as enjoyable and important as we are led to believe, or does ageing offer an opportunity to opt out of this relentless sexualization of all aspects of our lives? These questions will be addressed within the ensuing discussion and, in particular, it will be argued that attempts to 'explode' the myth of the asexual old age within the gerontological and health literatures, as well as the popular media, are actively creating a new form of stereotyping in its place, namely the myth of the 'sexy oldie'. The key messages underpinning this stereotype are that 'being sexual' is fundamental to mental and physical well-being at any age, but particularly as a means to stave off old age.

In addition, an analysis of the body of writing about sexuality and ageing within the gerontological and wider health literature reveals that these issues are typically situated within a particular, and very narrow context. For example, a romanticized notion of older people's sexuality is often presented – sex is talked about almost exclusively within the context of a loving, monogamous relationship. Many authors talk about 'making love', rather than sex – terminology that would rarely be used in relation to younger people. This conceptualization of later life sexuality leaves little room for issues such as sexual abuse, multiple sexual partnerships and non-heterosexuality, issues which reflect the experiences of many older people. Indeed, overall, later life sexuality tends to be presented very positively, as an almost mystical force which (always) promotes emotional and physical well-being.

Ageing, by contrast, is universally discussed in negative terms with a focus on age-related 'sexual dysfunctions' and health conditions that increase in prevalence with age (but do not define the experiences of most older people) such as cancer, heart disease and dementia. The role of medicine in helping older people to overcome the sexual problems that may result is made explicit. However, what is lacking is any recognition that the definitions of sexual problems and 'dysfunctions' unquestioningly adopted reflect dominant ideologies about sexuality (i.e. that sexual intercourse is the only 'true' sex), but not necessarily the beliefs and experiences of older people themselves.

This observation leads us to question the factors underpinning the myth of the 'sexy oldie'. Whilst presented in the literature, and often no doubt intended to be, a means to improve the quality of life of older people, writings that promote this vision must be situated within a wider socio-economic and cultural context. The focus of the last section of this chapter will be upon exploring this wider context and, in particular, elucidating the roles that medicalization, consumerism and the positive ageing movement are playing in the construction of the new stereotype of the 'sexy oldie'.

However, prior to this, key elements which it will be argued underpin the myth of the 'sexy oldie', will be explored through an analysis of the gerontological, health and wider popular literature. These include beliefs that: (1) sexuality is fundamental to healthy ageing; (2) sexual intercourse represents the sexual 'ideal' for older people; (3) expressing sexuality is about expressing love and is always a positive (and overwhelmingly heterosexual) experience; (4) ageing can, but need not cause sexual dysfunction, which can be 'fixed' by medical intervention, and (5) to be sexually attractive at any age you have to conform to a youthful notion of beauty (particularly if you are a woman).

The new myth (1): Expressing sexuality (preferably through sexual intercourse) is fundamental to healthy ageing

> After all this pessimism and simple inaccuracy it is a refreshing relief to learn that sex is good for older people.
>
> (Webb and Cordingley 1999: 485)

> Sexuality is now identified as a fundamental and natural need within everyone's life, regardless of age and physical state.
>
> (Pangman and Seguire 2000: 51)

> Sudden death during or after intercourse is rare and the benefits of intercourse, including ... gentle exercise and reduction of tension, outweigh the risks.
>
> (Webb and Cordingley 1999: 488)

As noted in the previous chapter, in contemporary society there has been an increasingly strong association made between good sex and good health. In a similar vein, there is a mounting body of scientific and popular literature proposing a straightforward link, between good sex and healthy ageing. Vincent, for example (2002: 248) writes in the academic journal *Sexual and Relationship Therapy* that: 'An absence of overall physical fitness, which, for some people, may include an active sex life, may predispose some women to risk of serious illnesses and disability in old age'. Starr and Weiner are more explicit about the need to remain sexually active at any age, claiming:

> Energy needs a place to go. When sexual energy is denied the outlet of behaviour that can provide sexual release, it goes into other areas. This process, called displacement, may result in illness – diarrhea, ulcers, heartburn, arthritis, neuralgia, and many other complaints familiar to older people.
>
> (1982: 10)

Similarly, to be able to *enjoy* sex when older some 'experts' argue that it is necessary to *never stop* having sex. Gurland and Gurland (1980: 72), for example, claim that 'The wisdom of beginning one's sex life early and remaining continuously in training in the interest of finishing it late, if at all, has been ... demonstrated.' In addition, Duffy proposes the 'use it or lose it' school of thought in relation to female sexuality and ageing:

> We know that we maintain physical function better when our bodies are in use as nature intended. Disuse can lead to disease and misuse to malfunction. Both men and women can maintain the integrity of their sexual organs when they are used. Health professionals should counsel clients on the benefits of remaining sexually active. Older women would thus be likely to experience greater vaginal lubrication and as rapidly as do younger women.
>
> (1998: 68)

Thereby a case is made for a *need* for adults, and in particular adult women, to be constantly sexual so they can have sex when older and hence 'ward off' old age. The assumption is always that having sex is fun, healthy and something that everybody not only *wants* to be doing, but ought to be doing.

Women are also being put under pressure to have sex as a means of remaining 'young and beautiful'. For example, a recent article from the online women's magazine 'handbag.com' cites consultant neuropsychologist Dr David Weeks (2003) and, in particular his conclusion from a 'decade-long study of more than 3500 people' that 'couples who have sex at least three times a week look 10 years younger than those of the same age who make love less frequently' (Richards 2003). He goes on to make the claim that this proves that 'pleasure from sex is a crucial factor in preserving youth, producing in women a human growth hormone that helps the process' http://www.handbag.com/relationship/sex/sexisgood.

But it doesn't stop there. If you don't manage to have enough sex to halt the ageing process altogether, then you are advised to still keep having it in order to promote your (declining) emotional and physical health. Matthias et al. (1997: 6), for example, argue that: 'Regardless of age, sexuality can be one of the human expressions that protects against alienation, coldness, and terror of an instrumental cost-accounting culture; a connection with the humanity in people for the celebration of being alive.' Similarly, Weg (1983: 45) while discussing sexuality and ageing argues: 'The intimacy and warmth often associated with sexual expression have significance beyond the pleasurable release of sexual tension – an important assertion of commitment of self and a reaffirmation of the connection with life itself.'

Taking this association between sex and health a step further are authors who claim that sex is not just 'good for you', but fundamental to your very humanity. For example, Gupta argues that 'sex and sexual needs are ... another physiologic necessity of human beings even in late life' (1990: 197). Framing sexuality as a 'necessity' seems to present older people with no option other than to be sexual. Doing so is presented not as a choice, but a responsibility. This is indicated in some of the discussions that have been held on how older women can meet their sexual 'needs', given the limited availability of older men. For example, Gurland and Gurland (1980: 69) conclude from their deliberations of this 'problem' that: 'The preponderance of women over men in older age groups, for example, invokes consideration of adaptive alternative lifestyles, such as lesbianism or marriage with younger men.' The message is that everybody should be sexually fulfilled to age healthily, even if it requires reconfiguring their sexual orientation. Indeed, sexual pleasure is afforded much higher priority than relationship satisfaction.

The notion that being sexually active, or more specifically having sexual intercourse, represents a human need which must be fulfilled has, unsurprisingly, been critiqued. Gannon, for example, eloquently argues:

> There is no evidence that sex in later life, or at any time of life, is a necessity – people who do not engage in sexual activity do not become sick, nor do they die. They may be unhappy because they wish to have sex and do not have a partner, but this is a social problem and not a biological or a medical problem and certainly does not apply to all older persons.
>
> (1999: 111)

Nevertheless, however rational this argument may seem, Gannon remains in a very small minority in critiquing the belief that sex is essential to healthy ageing. Indeed, later life sexual problems are firmly discussed within a medical, not a social context. What is further of concern is that this notion of sex as 'healthy', which underpins its perceived centrality to successful ageing, is led by 'expert' opinion bolstered by media interest rather than the experiences and beliefs of older people themselves. It also only allows for one model of 'normal' sexual expression, namely sexual intercourse.

The new myth (2): Sexual intercourse represents the sexual 'ideal' for all older people

Interviewer: So, ... to have sex without sexual intercourse ... does that happen at all in your relationship at the moment?
Interviewee: I don't think it does, no.
Interviewer: Right. So by that I mean, you know, either or both of you coming to orgasm without actually having intercourse. Or engaging in sexual activity in a prolonged sort of way.
Interviewee: Sorry? Coming to orgasm without having sexual intercourse? So how would that happen?

(Gavey et al. 1999: 41)

For older couples, being physically or spiritually close, showing tenderness or respect can be valued in such a way that intercourse is hardly missed.

(Hendricks and Hendricks 1978: 71)

The privileging of sexual intercourse over any other forms of sexual expression was discussed in the previous chapter and it is certainly a belief that pervades most thinking about sexuality and ageing. Indeed, the literature in this area devotes considerable time and energy to discussing how older people can make up for an inability to have sexual intercourse if health problems or erectile dysfunction makes this difficult. Other sexual behaviours are only discussed as a form of compensation if older people cannot have 'proper' sex. Such thinking reflects the taken-for-granted notion that sexual intercourse represents the 'best' and 'most healthy' sex. As discussed in the previous chapter, the hold that intercourse has over the popular imagination is unwavering. The first of the above quotations comes from a New Zealand study (Gavey et al. 1999), which looked at how heterosexuals account for intercourse and identified that, many male participants in particular, could see no other sexual alternatives.

Given how ingrained the idea that intercourse is the 'gold standard' of sexuality is, the inability of most of the sexuality and ageing literature to think beyond this is perhaps inevitable. However, in drawing together the findings of the above study, the authors conclude that there is a need to challenge the idea that intercourse represents the 'unquestioned and inevitable mark of "real" sex' and acknowledge it is 'one possibility among many' (Gavey et al. 1999: 63). While they present this shift as a means of reducing STI transmission, similar thinking could also be helpful in thinking about the centrality of sexual intercourse to understandings of sexuality and ageing.

A shift in thinking is particularly needed given the (very limited) evidence we have regarding how older people define and value sexuality. For example, in a recent study (Hinchliff and Gott 2004), we identified that a significant proportion of our married participants in their seventies had stopped having sexual intercourse for reasons such as experiencing erectile dysfunction, or their own or their partner's health problems. However, rather than representing a 'fate worse than death' as dominant ideologies would lead us to believe, this absence of penetrative sex was seen to be relatively straightforward to adjust to (even though it was missed). One participant, for example said that:

> As you get older I don't think a sexual relationship as such is as important as a love and cuddle ... we often have a cuddle and I mean I would never dream of walking out of the door without a cuddle and a kiss.
>
> (female participant, aged 72: quoted Hinchliff and Gott 2004: 603)

Furthermore, one older man also discussed how not being able to have intercourse did not mean that you could not have sex:

> As you get older you act differently and you adjust to your age, but I consider that a cuddle is sex ... intercourse doesn't take place as much when you're getting older, you're not able, but the desire to love someone is there, and love, it takes a different form. That's love when we are gardening together and doing things.
>
> (male participant, aged 74: quoted Hinchliff and Gott 2004: 604)

That older people may not automatically equate sex with intercourse is important and has not been recognized in the wider literature where it is still assumed that if you ask someone how often they have sex, what you are really asking them is how often they have intercourse.

A total focus on intercourse has also led to the marginalization of the aspects of sexuality that are not so amenable to definition, for example, body image and sexual attitudes and beliefs. Indeed, as will be seen in the next chapter, the coital focus taken in the sexuality and ageing literature has meant that all we know about older people's sexuality is frequency of sex (which is presumed to mean sexual intercourse). These more nebulous, and perhaps more interesting, aspects have been almost universally ignored and, crucially, older people themselves have rarely been asked about their understandings of sexuality.

As noted in the previous chapter, contemporary understandings of sexuality remain wedded not only to a coital, but to a reproductive norm – any forms of sexual expression that do not adhere to this can still be labelled 'deviant'. This is aptly exemplified by the heteronormativity (the belief that only heterosexual intercourse is normal) that continues to underpin distinctions drawn between normal and abnormal sexualities. While this assumption feeds into many discussions about sexuality, it particularly informs the ways in which sexuality and ageing are discussed. It is taken for granted by many that it is not only sexual intercourse, but heterosexual intercourse specifically, that is the norm for older people. For example, a study by Marsiglio and Donnelly (1991) only included married couples who were asked: "About how often did you and your husband/wife have sex during the past month?" However, at no point in the paper do they acknowledge that participants may have been having sex with someone other than their spouse and that not capturing this could be deemed a weakness of the study. The validity of this approach to explore sexual behaviours among younger people would be immediately questioned on these grounds. The assumption is that, for older people, sex equals heterosexual intercourse within marriage.

The new myth (3): Sex in later life is pleasurable and an expression of love

Implicit in the vast majority of discussions about sexuality and ageing and, in particular, the promotion of sex in old age is the taken-for-granted assumption that sex is a positive and pleasurable experience – something you (always) 'enjoy'. This is central even to the definitions of sexuality offered within the sexuality and ageing literature. For example, according to Hogan (1980: 3), sexuality includes: 'the quality of being human, all that we are as men and women ... encompassing the most intimate feelings and the deepest longings of the heart to find meaningful relationships'. Butler and Lewis (2002) again suggest that sexuality is more than a 'sex act', but rather represents an opportunity to express loyalty, passion, affection, esteem and affirmation of one's body and its functioning. One commentator goes so far as to state that, for older people, sex may be one of the few pleasures left (Duddle 1982).

Similarly, when sex in later life is discussed, it is often in terms of 'making love':

> Older love is gentler than young love. In old age the gymnastics of the twenty- or thirty-year-old will undoubtedly have given way to much smoother techniques of love-making. There is invariably more emphasis on caressing and cuddling and sexual play, rather than the hasty and spontaneous acts of a younger age group.
>
> (Sherman 1998: 5)

As this extract also clearly illustrates, later life sexuality is also often highly romanticized.

It could be hypothesized that this conflation between (heterosexual) sex and love makes older people's sexuality easier to accept. Issues such as non-heterosexual relationships, sexual risk-taking and the sexual abuse of older people get swept under the carpet because they do not conform to this romanticized and acceptable ideal. Commentators promoting later life sexuality, for example, consider sex to be 'fun, intimate, passionate, and a restorative force, bringing healing and a renewed energy for life' (Duddle 1982: 142). But sex can also be tedious, painful and abusive. Kleinschmidt (1997) notes that, while few estimates of the prevalence of sexual abuse of older people are available, they can be rendered vulnerable to such abuse by age-related physical and cognitive frailty. However, this is an area which is not addressed within the literature. Again, we can draw on feminist critiques which argue that the neglect of the dangerous side of sex (particularly for women) is ubiquitous within sexology, something attributed to a male-centred notion of sexuality to do with 'erotics' and not what makes people unhappy about sex in the real world (Tiefer 1995).

The new myth (4): Ageing causes sexual dysfunction and medical intervention is needed for older people to be sexually 'normal'

> In the light of all this [negative impact of ageing on sexuality], one might wonder how it is that so many older people manage to

remain sexually active. And a great many do, despite considerable physical impairment.

(Kaplan 1995: 299)

The therapeutic process helps them ... accommodate to the inevitable physical deficits of the aging process by "accentuating the (remaining) positives and decentuating the negatives".

(Kaplan 1995: 307)

In a society where sexual desire and performance have been deemed serious public health concerns (Laumann et al. 1999), and sexual normalcy is judged according to the ability to engage in sexual intercourse, growing older is seen to increase the risk of sexual dysfunction. The vast majority of literature in this area either implicitly or explicitly supports this belief through a focus on how to address barriers to engaging in sexual intercourse that increase in prevalence with ageing. A typical review of the sexuality and ageing literature will begin with the message that sex is crucial to quality of life for older people and then continue to detail all the ways in which ageing *negatively* affects sexuality. This will include specific genital malfunctions (notably erectile dysfunction, although increasing attention is being paid to 'female sexual dysfunction') as well as medical conditions which disproportionately affect older people, such as cardiovascular disease, diabetes, dementia and cancer. Non-coital forms of sexual expression may be briefly mentioned – typically cuddling or 'spiritual closeness'; (oral sex or mutual masturbation are not generally discussed in relation to this age cohort). However, this tends to be within the context that they can *compensate for* a reduced ability to have sexual intercourse (Hendricks and Hendricks 1978) as discussed previously. Finally, social and psychological factors will get a cursory look-in, particularly in relation to older women and the problems they are perceived to have in attracting older (male) partners.

Sexual dysfunctions are defined in relation to sexual intercourse, leading to 'genital performance during heterosexual intercourse ... [being viewed as] the essence of sexual functioning' (Tiefer 1995: 53). For example, a recent study of self-reported sexual problems classified these as follows: lack of interest in sex; anxiety about performance; unable to experience orgasm; premature orgasm; painful intercourse; unable to achieve or maintain an erection; and trouble lubricating (Mercer et al. 2003: Table BL1: 426). All of these are problems in meeting the ideal sexual end point, namely simultaneous orgasm during heterosexual intercourse (Hawkes 1996). In other words, if you do not desire intercourse, or cannot have intercourse satisfactorily (which includes having an orgasm), then you have a sexual 'problem'. Whether you consider you have a sexual problem or not appears largely irrelevant.

Against this background, it is unsurprising that older people are deemed 'dysfunctional'. Increases in the incidence of erectile dysfunction and vaginal dryness with age can make sexual intercourse problematic for some and this is certainly stressed in the literature. For example, Bancroft argues that 'there is an undoubted decline in the sexuality of both men and women with advancing years' (1983: 282), and exemplifies this by citing figures showing evidence that older people report lower 'levels' of interest in and rates of sexual intercourse than they experienced when they were younger. He acknowledges that this 'catalogue of decline may seem gloomy' (1983: 288).

However, his list of sexual problems which accompany ageing is perhaps not as gloomy as that provided by a special edition of the journal *Sexual and Relationship Therapy* (2002) on 'Sex and intimacy in older people', which includes five papers on sexuality within the context of mental health problems (the implication being that all older people are either battling depression or dementia which has an important, negative effect on their sex life). Other papers focus on topics as cheerful as '[sexual] health *challenges* for older women' (Vincent 2002: 241) and the negative effects on female sexuality of the menopause and (apparently) related conditions (including cancer). Indeed, in nearly everything written about sexuality and ageing, a process of inevitable decline from a youthful norm is invoked, with the health problems and age-related physiological changes that may render sexual intercourse problematic discussed.

Having established that sexual dysfunction is age-related, the role for health professionals in 'improving the sexual expression and fulfilment of the elderly person' (Gurland and Gurland 1980: 67) is made apparent. Kessel, for example, in the UK journal *Age and Ageing*, aimed at geriatricians, states that: 'Professionals should advise that sex is good for you and orgasm achieved by masturbation may relieve anxiety and promote well being' (2001: 122). Similarly, Schlesinger (1996: 125) argues: 'Sexuality should be viewed as a birth to death phenomenon. Just as health care providers assist the elderly to walk, eat, exercise and have regular bowel movements, so too should they assist them to be sexual human beings.' The (ageist) assumption that older people cannot be sexual without professional assistance is discussed further below.

The new myth (5): To be sexually attractive at any age you need to conform to a youthful standard of beauty (particularly if you are a woman)

> [Jane Fonda] has a great body, an over-40 body that offers hope and promise. Along with each book and tape comes convincing evidence that it's possible ... to remain beautiful and sexy in midlife.
>
> (Levin 1987: 27)

> Comparing when I was 21 and 41, the amount of attention I attracted when I entered a room was as different as, respectively, a famous actor at the height of their career and an unemployed cleaning lady.
>
> (cited James 2003
> http://observer.guardian.co.uk/magazine/story/0,11913,1041284,000.html)

> Outward bodily signs ... [are] mirrors of morality, ... So too, our bodies are mirrors of mortality.
>
> (Blaikie 1999: 86)

In the previous chapter, the increasing trend to conflate an inherent sexuality with an exterior 'sexiness', or beauty, was discussed. It was argued that, to be perceived as sexual, older people, and older women in particular, have to conform to contemporary youthful standards of sexual attractiveness. Not only is the older body not deemed sexually attractive, it is held up as the very antithesis of sexuality and beauty. It represents the physical manifestation of an asexual end point to be avoided at any costs, at any age.

Resisting the physical ravages of old age is a crucial element of the 'sexy oldie' stereotype, particularly in relation to the ways in which ageing and sexuality are increasingly understood in contemporary culture. Indeed, those older people who are held up as examples of how ageing and sexuality need not be incompatible are invariably those who 'look good for their age'. As such, they do not challenge the understanding that old age cannot be sexy, but rather actively reinforce it. As Sontag (1979) argues:

> They are admired precisely because they are exceptions, because they have managed (at least so it seems in photographs) to outwit nature. Such miracles, exceptions made by nature (with the help of art and social privilege), only confirm the rule, because what makes these women seem beautiful to us is precisely that they do not look their real age. Society allows no place in our imagination for a beautiful old woman who does look ... old. http://www.mediawatch.com/sontag.html

She also (rightly) identifies that these women tend to have access to amounts of money to spend on maintaining their youthful beauty that are beyond the means of most.

However, it is not seen as enough to merely spend the money, buy the lotions and make-up and have the surgery. The end result also has to look 'natural'. If it is *obvious* that an older person has worked hard to achieve this youthful veneer, then that hard work becomes invalidated. For example, for older women, wearing too much make-up, dressing inappropriately youthfully and having obvious cosmetic surgery, can all hold you up as an object of ridicule – 'mutton dressed as lamb', an 'old slapper'. Although older men are not subjected to the same pressures, trying to disguise grey hair, or even worse wearing a toupee, can similarly render you ridiculous.

Returning to the issue of gender, it is certainly true that Susan Sontag's 'double standard' of ageing is alive and well in the twenty-first century in that physical ageing continues to disenfranchise and desexualize women in a way that it does not men (although the gap is narrowing). As such, the following discussions of the implications of sexual unattractiveness and concomitant asexuality relate in the main to women and have been articulated in the main by feminist authors.

The implications of sexual disenfranchisement as a result of an ageing body can be profound, again particularly for women. Travis et al. (2000: 237) argue that 'Beauty is considered to be a fundamental quality in women', a quality which emanates from the association between bodily control, self-control and moral superiority. Whilst the traditional linkage between the disciplining of the body and religious growth holds little sway within our increasingly secular society, a 'new ascetism' or 'New Puritanism' (Turner

1984; Kilwein 1989) has emerged which attaches similar moral value to maintaining a fit and healthy body. For women, it is not just a fit body, but a beautiful fit body, which signifies an inherent 'goodness' of character. If women do not exert the self-control needed to present this beautiful body, then they are not only viewed as lazy, but even potentially as mentally ill (Travis et al. 2000). The implication is that 'It is only acceptable to be older if the woman continues to look 30' (2000: 251).

However, 'letting yourself go' does not merely sexually disenfranchise you in the eyes of society (and maybe your own eyes as well) it is also socially disenfranchising. The quote at the beginning of this section is illustrative of the invisibility of older women worldwide (Weil 2001). Moreover, when older women are made visible, the resulting images tend not to be flattering. Within literature and myth, for example, representations of old women are almost universally negative, as 'crone', 'hag', or 'witch' (Rotosky and Brown Travis 2000). Comparative terms do not exist for older men.

Overall, therefore, to maintain perceived 'goodness', social worth, social visibility and particularly sexuality, it is necessary to minimize the physical effects of ageing. Moreover, given these associations, so doing is presented not as a choice, but as a responsibility. As Greer argues:

> There is no point at which the middle-aged woman can make plain her opting out of certain kinds of social interaction. She has a duty to go on 'being attractive' no matter how fed up she is with the whole business. She is not allowed so say 'Now I shall let myself go'; letting herself go is a capital offence.
>
> (1991: 38)

How have we arrived at the stereotype of the 'sexy oldie'?

Having identified the emergence of a new form of stereotyping, it is important to explore those factors that are promoting this shift in the ways in which ageing and sexuality are understood. Doing so will be the focus of the current section and, in particular, three key trends will be examined: (1) the medicalization of (ageing) sexuality; (2) the 'positive ageing' movement; and (3) the 'baby boomer' generation.

Medicalization of ageing sexuality

As argued in the previous chapter, the influence of medicine upon what we think of as sexuality has been profound (Weeks 1986). Moreover, the case was made that this influence is becoming ever more pervasive and, in particular, is extending into the realms of sexual performance and sexual pleasure to the extent that the sexual fulfilment of a population has become viewed as a major 'public health' concern (Laumann et al. 1999). This shift in thinking about sexuality has been partly brought about by the emergence of erectile dysfunction and, more recently, female sexual dysfunction as definable medical disorders which are said to affect a large proportion of the population and, it is claimed, increase in prevalence with age.

Tiefer (1986) outlines the ways in which male sexual performance became increasingly medicalized from the 1980s onwards, focusing specifically upon the growth of a new medical specialty of 'male sexual dysfunction' within urology and a related conceptual shift in understanding erectile problems. Not only was 'impotence' (something no man would readily identify with) repackaged as 'erectile dysfunction', but urologists stressed the vascular, physiological basis of the condition, rather than the psychological factors which had previously been seen as the primary underlying cause (Katz and Marshall 2003). Moreover, this 'pursuit of the perfect penis' (Tiefer 1986: 1), bolstered by drug company money and media interest, led to urologists becoming the definers and healers of masculinity (Hellstrom 1999). Indeed, a medical response was seen as the only option for what was increasingly seen as an organic condition with profound psychosocial consequences (Katz and Marshall 2003). By the time the FDA approved sildenifil citrate as an oral medication for erectile dysfunction in 1998, taking a pill to 'solve' erectile dysfunction was seen as a logical, or even the *only*, logical response and medicine's regulation of male sexuality was hence cemented.

Given the commercial success of Viagra, as well as its profound impact upon public beliefs about sexuality, the search for a female alternative was inevitable. By 1997, the eminent US urologist Irwin Goldstein was arguing that 'female sexual dysfunction' would become a significant focus for urology and drawing equivalencies between male and female sexualities, claiming that: 'We think [diminished blood flow to the vagina] is equivalent to vascolgenic impotence in men' (Bankhead 1997: 1). In 1998 it was Goldstein again who produced a consensus statement which, drawing heavily upon the language of the *Diagnostic and Statistical Manual* (*DSM-IV*), produced by the American Psychiatric Association (2003), pulled off a 'tactical coup' (Tiefer 2001: 68) in defining both male and female sexual dysfunctions as medical, not psychological disorders. Interestingly, he also identified them as disorders of ageing (see, for example, Park et al. 1997; Moynihan 2003a). All that was needed now was some understanding of the epidemiology of the condition and this was provided in a 1999 paper published in the *Journal of the American Medical Association* (Laumann et al. 1999), which claimed a prevalence of female sexual dysfunction of 43 per cent among American women over the age of 18. However, this figure remains highly controversial as it defined a dysfunction as experiencing only one of seven sexual problems during the past month. Indeed, whichever way one looks at it, defining nearly half of the female populations of the UK and the USA as sexually abnormal appears problematic.

By 2001, interest in, and awareness of, 'female sexual dysfunction' were evidenced in the huge number of responses generated by an article in the *British Medical Journal* arguing that this was in fact a condition invented by drug companies to boost their profits, rather than a 'real illness' experienced by 'real women' (Moynihan 2003a). Hundreds of letters were sent from both sides of the debate. Women with sexual problems wrote in to complain that Moynihan's attack invalidated their own experience and distress. Professionals both refuted and supported his claims ('I think there is a dissatisfaction and perhaps disinterest among a lot of women, but that doesn't mean they have a disease': Leiblum, cited in Moynihan 2003a: 46). Many academic psychologists and sociologists supported his position, arguing that women's sexual problems are not only highly heterogeneous in cause and effect, but may potentially have more to do with sexual relationships than a disease or dysfunction model. While it was clear that no consensus could ever be reached, the extreme interest and passion the debate generated exemplified the highly political and endlessly fascinating nature of sexuality and, particularly medicine's role therein, in the early twenty-first century.

These are important trends to chart because they are having a profound influence upon the involvement of medicine in the understanding and 'management' of ageing sexuality. Indeed, both erectile dysfunction and female sexual dysfunction are said to increase in prevalence with age. For example, it has been estimated that a man aged 70 is three times more likely to have 'complete' erectile dysfunction than a man aged 40 (Glossman et al. 1999) and studies to date indicate that between 20 per cent and 52 per cent of older men have experienced erectile dysfunction within the past year (Simons and Carey 2001). Older men are also more likely to have their erectile dysfunction attributed to an organic cause related to 'normal ageing' (Schiavi 1999). Similarly, it has been suggested that female sexual dysfunction is 'age-related and progressive' so that older women have more sexual difficulties than younger ones (Berman and Bassuk 2002: 111). Moreover, Schiavi (1999) proposes that age-related physiological changes in sexual functioning render both older women and men more vulnerable, sexually, to psychosocial stresses.

In addition, younger people are increasingly being identified as markets for drugs that prevent the onset of age-related sexual dysfunctions. For example, Irwin Goldstein claimed recently that he was a 'strong believer' in taking Viagra on a daily basis to 'prevent impotence'. His belief is predicated on the grounds that 'If you would like to be sexually active in five years time, take a quarter of a pill a night – we have data to show that will facilitate and prolong nocturnal erections' (cited in Moynihan 2003b: 9). Why you *need* nocturnal erections is not addressed. Similarly, women are increasingly being sold the 'use it or lose it' model of sexual activity as discussed earlier in this chapter, whereby stopping having sexual intercourse is seen as a precursor to a sexually dysfunctional later life. Furthermore, it won't be long before a suitable medication for preventing the onset of female sexual dysfunction is made available. As Goldstein (2003) argues: 'There is a generation of women getting older who started the sexual revolution ... Osteoporosis is a natural part of aging, but that doesn't mean we don't keep people from trying to break their hips.' http://www.cbsnews.com/stories/2004/05/03/eveningnews/main615320.shtml

The underlying message, therefore, is that 'normal ageing' can, but need not, cause 'sexual dysfunctions' which are amenable to both medical classification and medical treatment. Ultimately, this 'refashioning of sexual dysfunctions as age-related organic diseases, yet not necessarily organic consequences of aging, consigns us to always think of bodies as unfinished and puts all men and all women potentially at risk' (Katz and Marshall 2003: 12–13). Any loss of sexual desire or sub-optimal performance of sexual intercourse at any age is labelled 'abnormal' and 'unhealthy', to the extent that all adults are expected to be sexually active and, crucially, sexually fulfilled.

The 'positive ageing' movement

Another contributory factor to the new view of later life sexuality represented by the 'sexy oldie' has undoubtedly been the 'positive ageing' movement. This reconceptualization of ageing as an affirmative, rather than negative, experience has been in evidence since the 1970s as a means to challenge the ageism inherent in society (Bytheway 1995). The central tenet of this thinking is that, to improve quality of life for older people, there is a need to reframe the ways in which we think about the ageing process. As the Positive Ageing Foundation of Australia states: 'positive ageing is a new way of thinking about growing old that focuses on the opportunities and challenges that this period in the lifespan can bring' (http://www.positiveageing. com.au/PAFA_Research.htm). Such thinking has also been boosted by the claims of anti-ageing medicine whose mission is to detect, prevent, treat and reverse age-related disease (American Academy of Anti-Aging Medicine 2003). It is symbolized by the image of the 90-year-old marathon runner and the 80-year-old body builder – old, healthy bodies taking part in traditionally youthful pursuits. These images and messages have also fed into media representations of later life. As Blaikie notes: 'In the popular media, a vision which pictures old people as a passive and pathological problem group characterised by dependency has been partially eclipsed by "positive ageing" messages about the hedonistic joys of leisured retirement' (1999: 15).

At first glance, there seems little to criticize in the 'positive ageing' movement. Surely viewing ageing as not inevitably leading to physical, mental and socio-economic decline can only be a good thing? However, look further. What implications does such thinking have for the lives of 'ordinary' older men and women? As Blaikie states: 'Ironically, positive ageing has produced its own tyrannical imperative: unless you work at being "liberated" from chronological destiny, you are less than normal' (1999: 209). He goes on to state: 'These practices of positive ageing effectively transform physical and mental problems associated with biological ageing into social deviance, which, in turn, becomes evidence of clinical pathology' (1999: 209). Such thinking is also imbued with paternalistic overtones. In the words of Byethway: 'It is ... not difficult to see in this anti-ageing positivism an element of knowing what's best for them, believing we know all the answers, blaming others for their ignorance and misery, and seeking to save them through exhortation and example' (1995: 128).

It is certainly not difficult to view the 'sexy oldie' as a by-product of a positive ageing movement which, while intending to combat ageism, may unwittingly have also achieved the opposite effect. Indeed, the paternalism which Bytheway invokes is characteristic of the perceived role of health professionals in later life sexual health management in much of the literature, namely to 'assist' older people to be sexual (something they obviously need help with). Similarly, the need to work at resisting age-related changes in sexual function also forms part of a larger project to 'liberate' yourself from chronological age entirely. If you do not succeed, you are deemed a failure.

The 'baby boomer' generation

> Each cohort of retired persons is the product of a particular
> generation and each possess a unique as well as a common culture.
>
> (Gilleard and Higgs 2000: 44)

> Sexual intercourse began
> In nineteen sixty-three
> (Which was rather late for me)
> Between the end of the Chatterley ban
> And the Beatles' first LP.
>
> (Philip Larkin, 'Annus Mirabilis', 1974)

The 'baby boomers' who once defined 'youth culture' are now themselves entering later life and in so doing 'confounding ideas of what it means to be old' (Gilleard and Higgs 2000: 9). In particular, while it is certainly important not to overplay homogeneity by age, it is likewise necessary to remember that this is a generation socialized in a time when contemporary culture, and particularly the role of sex therein, changed radically. Indeed, the uncoupling of sex from reproduction (Hawkes 1996) through the availability of the oral contraceptive pill and a related relaxation of sexual mores, particularly in relation to the acceptability of heterosexual intercourse outside marriage, meant that sex became an acceptable, and fashionable, leisure pursuit for both men and women. Notably it became a defining part of a new, autonomous teenage sub-culture created and perpetuated by the cinema and a media-created image of how young people ought to behave (Schofield 1965). Sex also served as a point of differentiation between the new youth culture and an older generation and, particularly, as a means for younger people to develop an identity and lifestyle distinct from their parents (Hawkes 1996).

In addition, the babyboomer generation gave birth to the 'pop' culture which, it is claimed (Gilleard and Higgs 2000), destabilized the traditional site of social and economic weight, namely the value system expressed through the lives of middle-aged 'upper middle-class' men. A new consumer society emerged, headed up by pop stars and fashion photographers, and fuelled by the increasing availability of new leisure technologies. This desire for the new 'stimulated economic growth, expanded markets at home and abroad and consolidated a mass consumer society where young adults could establish a position for themselves in direct (and profitable) conflict with "the establishment"' (Gilleard and Higgs 2000: 63). Ultimately, this fostered both the centrality of youth to contemporary culture and the centrality of consumption to identity formation.

That this age cohort appears to be particularly fearful of ageing is therefore unsurprising. Indeed, many are happy to spend vast amounts on maintaining a youthful, sexualized veneer, a trend which also fits with the increased responsibility afforded to individuals, rather than the state, in maintaining health, wealth and well-being at all life stages (Gilleard and Higgs 2000). Gilleard and Higgs also claim that they are the first generation who can actively choose how they age:

Only in the late twentieth century has the idea emerged that human agency can be exercised over how ageing will be expressed and experienced. The assumption that individuals can choose the manner in which they wish to mark out their lives is a radical break with the past.

(2000: 3)

Indeed, the increased resources available to some older people mean that, increasingly, choices can be made about appearance and behaviour in later life. Moreover, the lifestyles they can purchase have come to define majority expectations of ageing and old age. In particular, securing the means to minimize unwelcome age-related changes in the body, such as grey hair and wrinkles, have become seen as more than a choice, but a necessity. Appearing old represents failure.

The next section will explore the ways in which the (perceived) consumer power of the babyboomer generation is increasingly being harnessed by marketing strategies that have recognized the economic benefits of pushing 'age-resisting' technologies (Gilleard and Higgs 2000). Of particular concern will be the implications such marketing has for sexuality and ageing, where the key question to be addressed relates to the extent to which it is contributing towards the belief that sexual fulfilment in later life is a 'need'.

Sex, consumerism and the 'gold in grey'

With increasing longevity and the coming of the "age wave," adulthood (not youth) is becoming the new marketplace epi-center. Learn about the core consumer needs and dreams driven by the new adult lifestages including: empty-nesting, grandparenthood, singlehood, and retirement, and discover the adult-oriented boom products and services of tomorrow.

(Ken Dytchwald, http://www.agewave.com/lifecourse.shtml)

Current efforts to develop and capture the aging market may sometimes have the effect of creating needs where none exist ... and especially diverting attention from the needs of low income elderly people.

(Minkler 1991: 82)

In this debate, the economic potential of exploiting both sexuality and older people must be recognized. The old adage that 'sex sells' is more of a truism now than it ever has been, but what is new is the increasing recognition of the 'gold in grey' (Minkler 1991). As Gilleard and Higgs (2000: 9) acknowledge, not only are more people living into retirement than ever before, but they also have 'more resources through which to shape their retirement, enabling a greater engagement with contemporary "lifestyle culture"'. This is highly relevant to sexuality, given its focus upon the maintenance of the body, and recognition of the marketing potential of promoting 'healthy ageing' of which, it has been argued, sexual intercourse is increasingly seen as a part.

Indeed, marketing companies are growing ever more aware of the economic benefits to be reaped from the affluent section of the older population. As the website 'the maturemarket.com' acknowledges: 'big industry, from sports to pharmaceuticals and cosmetics ... are designing and marketing totally new products tailored to the specific needs and wants of baby boomers, and the new model of adulthood they have created'. The identification of the role older people are playing in actively 'creating' a new postmodern lifecourse where age divisions are blurred is crucial. From this perspective, older people are *empowering themselves* to resist old age – the age-resisting technologies are produced as a response to this need. As such, the marketing agencies could be positively encouraged for challenging ageist assumptions which have traditionally marginalized older consumers.

However, is there not a danger that the economic potential of 'gold in grey' (Minkler 1991) could lead to the creation of needs where they did not previously exist? As Estes has convincingly argued (1979: 238):

> The social needs of the elderly ... are defined in ways compatible with the ... economy. The effect ... is to transform these needs into government-funded and industry-developed commodities for specific economic markets, commodities that are then consumed by the elderly.

While the 'ageing enterprise' to which she refers was discussed with particular reference to the USA, and is certainly most in evidence there, there is certainly no doubt that, as with so many things, where the USA leads, Britain follows.

So what does this mean for sexuality and ageing? First, it raises the question of the extent to which the 'need' for sexual fulfilment at any age represents a real need experienced by real people. As discussed previously in relation to the medicalization of sexuality, the economic benefits of promoting this way of thinking are enormous. Tiefer (2000) argues that pharmaceutical companies increasingly wish to develop drugs which are not disease-specific, but will appeal to large segments of the population. Therefore, 'An aging population presents new opportunities for the development of such drugs to offset the maladies of *loss* related to normal aging' (Katz and Marshall 2003: 11), including sexual loss. In addition, the way in which the cosmetics industry has promoted the importance of maintaining a sexualized (youthful) appearance as a means to increase women's (and increasingly men's) anxieties about ageing and, hopefully, their willingness to invest in products that resist it, is well known. Overall, therefore, it can certainly be argued that marketing companies and private economic interests have helped foster contemporary fears of an asexual old age and the need to resist this by remaining a 'sexy oldie'. Indeed, these markets seem only to be limited by the economic resources of the new oldies because:

> There is no escape ... since one cannot rationally choose to decline. In fact, individuals skilled in the exercise of consumer choice must choose to be posthumanly and timelessly functional and do so by embracing the benevolent promise of modern technology. Sexual function, like physical

fitness more generally, has become central to contemporary conceptions of the good life.

(Katz and Marsall 2003: 13)

Conclusion

This chapter has proposed that a new form of stereotyping is increasingly framing understandings of sexuality and ageing, namely the 'sexy oldie'. Emerging not only within the gerontological and wider health and social science literature, but also within the popular imagination, this conceptualization of later life sexuality is typically discussed as a 'good thing' which 'liberates' older people from the myth of the asexual old age. However, it has been argued that, while at first glance a seemingly positive trend, this new way of thinking about sexuality in relation to older people demands critical discussion. Not only does it present older people with little choice but to remain sexual if they want to remain socially engaged, but it also leaves little room for their own attitudes, experiences and behaviours. Crucially, as with all stereotyping, it leaves no room for diversity.

Moreover, while presented as attempts to sexualize old age, it seems apparent that the main messages that emerge from this body of work actually propose a sexualization of an extended middle age because the strategies presented to older people to remain sexual reflect and reinforce youth-centred definitions of sexuality. For example, appearing sexual requires adhering to youthful notions of beauty and, through whatever means available, eliminating signs of ageing which do not conform with this, such as wrinkles and grey hair. Similarly, remaining 'sexually active' is defined in terms of continuing to engage in sexual intercourse, something that is likely to assume less importance with ageing (Gott and Hinchliff 2003a), but is still sold as the taken-for-granted pinnacle of sexual experience. There is no room for older people to define how they view sexuality and, effectively, the notion that old age can never be sexual is reinforced – older people can be sexual only if they adhere to global (youthful) ideas about what this is. Moreover, older people have not escaped the increasingly explicit linkages between (good) sex and (good) health to the extent that sexual fulfilment is seen as a fundamental human right and ensuring it, an individual responsibility. The exit from the relentlessly sexualized world that ageing has the potential to provide is shut off. When viewed in this light, attempts to sexualize old age are not as liberating as they may at first appear.

Furthermore, while seemingly empowering to older people, these new messages about ageing and sexuality have not just emerged to improve the quality of later life. Medicine is increasingly claiming sexuality, including sexual pleasure, as its own domain and issues of medical territorialism and drug company profits must be considered in any discussion of the sexualization of later life. Indeed, acknowledging the relationship between the recognition of the potential older consumer market and the identification/ creation of older people's needs is crucial. In addition, active sexuality may be fundamental to the healthy and positive ageing movements, but is this model of ageing more prescriptive than liberating? Finally, does the characterization of babyboomers as the leisured, sexually voracious retired merely serve to mask the real needs of socially disenfranchised older people, of which there are many today in the UK?

Indeed, overall the failure of the vast majority of writing about sexuality and ageing to take on board the heterogeneity of older people is striking. Talk of sexuality as a prop to fuel consumption reminds us that the ability to consume varies markedly among older people – Gannon (1999: 124) argues, for older people 'who are struggling to survive, sexuality is simply irrelevant'. Gender differences have been identified in this discussion and will receive further attention, as will some of the other social divisions which can be drawn between people of the same age, such as sexual orientation and living circumstances. While the first two chapters of this book have explored the myths and stereotypes which typify contemporary understandings of sexuality and ageing, the next three chapters will explore what we actually know about how older people themselves in all their diversity define, value and express their sexuality.

PART II

Focusing upon older people's experiences of sexuality and ageing

What do we 'know' about sexuality and ageing?

A new look at the literature

The present study is designed as a first step in the accumulation of a body of scientific fact that may provide the bases for sounder generalizations about the sexual behaviour of certain groups and, some day, even of our American population as a whole.

(Kinsey et al. 1948: 34)

Sexological writings are frequently so preoccupied with the quantification of data regarding sexual behaviours and functions that they rarely pause to consider how or why sexuality might resist the structures of categorization that sexual science multiplies at an exponential rate.

(Bristow 1997: 15)

Introduction: The 'usual suspects', Kinsey and beyond

A typical overview of the sexuality and ageing literature will begin with Kinsey et al. (1948, 1953) and continue to explore the work of Masters and Johnson (1966, 1970) and then later (US) surveys of later life sexual behaviour. This chapter may not at first seem to be departing from that traditional model, as the 'usual suspects' will again be discussed. However, a much more critical perspective will be adopted than that taken to date. Indeed, while previous reviews have highlighted problems with discrete aspects of methodology, the current review will critique the entire philosophy behind this body of work. In particular, it will be argued that the 'sexological model' (Tiefer 2000) which informs the majority of this research, limits the contribution it can make to understandings of later life sexuality.

The present review is not comprehensive. It covers studies which have had the most significant impact upon understandings of sexuality and ageing,

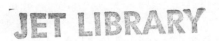
JET LIBRARY

although small-scale studies are addressed where their approach departs from that traditionally adopted. In the final section of the chapter, literature will be presented which explores issues of sexual attractiveness, 'beauty' and body image among older people. Although such work is rarely framed as 'sexuality research', it is important to consider it in this context if we are to move from a narrow, coital-focused view of sexuality and ageing. These discussions will provide the background to the next chapter, which will present findings from one of the first qualitative studies to be published in the UK, exploring older people's beliefs about, and experiences of, later life sexuality.

Kinsey et al.: Sexual behaviour in the human male and female

Alfred Kinsey was a zoologist by training and his principal expertise, prior to taking on the task of mapping human sexual behaviour in America, was the taxonomic classification of gall wasps. While this may seem a trivial aside, it was in fact fundamental to the entire methodological approach adopted in those landmark studies of sexual behaviour in the human male and female. Indeed, he felt strongly that the taxonomic method, which had served him so well in his studies of insects, was the 'scientific' approach needed to name, describe and classify human sexual behaviours in such a way as to establish norms of behaviour for entire populations. Moreover, he firmly believed that understanding human sexuality, like understanding wasp behaviour, involved understanding biology. He argues that:

> The difficulties that might be encountered in undertaking such a study promised to be greater than those involved in studying insects. The gathering of the human data would involve the learning of new techniques in which human personalities would be the obstacles to overcome and human memories would be the instruments whose use we would have to master.
>
> (Kinsey et al. 1948: 9–10)

However, having mastered these instruments, the implication was that the essence of human sexuality would be uncovered, classified and thereby understood.

In order to arrive at these 'scientific facts' of human sexual behaviour, lengthy interviews were conducted with 5300 men aged 10–80 years and 5940 women aged up to 90 years. The specific interests of the research team, and hence the focus of the interviews, are evident in the two resulting books which compile the research findings according to types, frequencies, sources and socio-demographic correlates of 'sexual outlet'. 'Sexual outlet' was defined as orgasm resulting from masturbation, nocturnal emissions, petting to climax, pre-marital intercourse, marital intercourse, homosexual outlet and (who can forget) animal contacts.

In relation to later life sexuality, Kinsey, Pomeroy and Martin (1948) state that the dominant assumptions about sexuality and ageing among biologists and health care professionals at the time when their study was initiated was that males reach a peak of sexual 'capacity' in their thirties and forties, beyond which point such capacity 'drops away abruptly into the inactivity and complete impotence of old age' (1948: 222). However, within their sample of males aged 10–80 years, the authors identified no such 'abrupt cut-off', but rather a gradual decline in all measures of 'sexual outlet'. They conclude that they do not have enough evidence to isolate factors associated with this decline, but postulate that it could be related to physiological factors, psychological factors, reduced availability of partners, or preoccupation with 'social or business functions' (1948: 229). Presumably this decline relates to individuals under the age of 80, because they later conclude that 'most males, but not all of them, would become [impotent] if they all lived into their eighties' (1948: 237). However, the confidence of these conclusions, and their subsequent impact upon understandings of sexuality and ageing, must be questioned, given that they were based on a sample which included only four males in their eighties. Indeed, overall, only 10 per cent (542) of the male sample was over 50 and a very small proportion over 60 (131 aged 60–69; 37 aged 70–79; and 4 aged 80), which tells us something about the importance Kinsey placed upon later life sexuality.

The study of female sexual behaviour was initiated in the same research centre five years later (Kinsey et al. 1953). Again, few older women were included (214 over 50; 46 over 60; and 10 over 70), although findings significant to contemporary understandings of female sexuality and ageing were reported. These included the conclusion that: 'Among females the median frequencies of those sexual activities, which are not dependent upon the male's initiation of socio-sexual contacts, remain more or less constant from the late teens into the fifties and sixties' (1953: 715). Indeed, they claim that 'one of the tragedies' of marriage is that men are more sexually interested than women when younger, while by the age of 50 it is women who are more sexually motivated than men. They relate this to the impact of 'physiologic' ageing upon male sexual capacity, but not female sexual capacity. By examining frequency of masturbation and 'nocturnal dreams to orgasm', they conclude that 'the female frequencies rise gradually to their maximum point and then stay more or less on a level until after fifty-five or sixty years of age' (1953: 353). The potential to investigate what happens to women after this point was obviously hampered by the very small numbers of participants over 60, although the authors seem confident in their conclusion that 'Individuals who have reached old age are no longer as capable of responding [sexually] as they were at an earlier age' (1953: 715).

The main criticisms that have been levelled at Kinsey's work in relation to later life sexuality have focused in the main upon the small numbers of older people included in both the male and female studies, although discussions have also highlighted that drawing conclusions regarding interactions between ageing and sexuality from cross-sectional data is problematic because it does not allow for the confounding nature of cohort effects to be explored (George and Weiler 1981). However, the overall approach to studying sexual behaviour that Kinsey and colleagues established has not been critiqued within the sexuality and ageing literature and, indeed, has set a methodological precedent for most subsequent research undertaken in this area.

As such, critically examining these studies is important and, so doing, identifies more fundamental challenges that can be levelled against this work. Of particular concern are the authors' beliefs that: (1) sexuality is a biological 'essence' (Tiefer 1995); (2) sex consists mainly of those acts related to intercourse; (3) orgasm, particularly for men, is the 'most precise and scientific indicator of a sexual experience' (Bancroft 1998: e); (4) gender differences in sexual behaviours are 'natural'; (5) the notion that sex is healthy; and (6) the idea that the best way to understand sexuality is to classify particular sexual behaviours. These are ideas that were discussed and deconstructed in the previous chapters and will receive further attention later in the book. They do not therefore warrant extensive further discussion at this point, suffice to say that, when explored empirically and philosophically, they are revealed as deeply problematic. However, as will be seen, they continue to underpin sexuality and ageing research to this day.

Masters and Johnson (1966, 1970)

Masters and Johnson initiated the next landmark research project which had a significant impact upon beliefs about sexuality and ageing, although again not many older people were included. In their two books, *Human Sexual Response* (1966) and *Human Sexual Inadequacy* (1970), the authors aimed to explore the nature and causes of possible sexual dysfunction at all ages through addressing the following research question: 'What physical reactions develop as the human male and female respond to effective sexual stimulation?" (How 'effective' sexual stimulation can be defined was unclear.) A sample of 382 female and 312 male participants aged 18–89 years old was recruited and subjected to a series of laboratory tests, including 'artificial coition' (Masters and Johnson 1966) where female participants were penetrated by electrically powered plastic penises.

Data derived from these participants was used to develop the most far-reaching legacy of Masters and Johnson's work – the 'Human Sexual Response Cycle' (HSRC). The HSRC will be familiar to most, if not by that name, in the way in which it divides human sexual response into four discrete phases: (1) the excitement phase; (2) the plateau phase; (3) the orgasmic phase; and (4) the resolution phase. This model, which is resolutely grounded in biology, continues to underpin contemporary beliefs about sexual response, as well as medical classifications of sexual dysfunctions. However, it has come under significant critique. For example, it has been highlighted that research participants had to have previous orgasmic experience during intercourse to be recruited into the study, as well as to be of 'higher intelligence'. As such, it has been claimed that 'the discovery of the HSRC ... [was] a self-fulfilling prophecy, with the research subjects selected to compress diversity' (Tiefer 1995: 44).

To explore 'geriatric sexual response', 34 women and 39 men over the age of 50 were subjected to 'concentrated investigation' over four years (Masters and Johnson 1966: 223). The authors acknowledge that older participants were even more highly selected than the remainder of the sample, given the difficulties of enrolling this age group into the study. Moreover, they write that the small sample means that they are only able to 'suggest clinical impression rather than to establish biologic fact' (1966: 223) (as with Kinsey, they obviously considered the essence of sexuality to lie in biology).

Perhaps the most important clinical impression they offer in relation to later life sexuality regards their conclusion that physiological ageing processes do not preclude sexual activity in later life, and that ageing may even bring potential *benefits* to sexual response – as radical an idea today as it was at the time. For example, they claim that 'many a woman develops renewed interest in her husband and in the physical maintenance of her own person, and has described a "second honeymoon" in her early 50s' (Masters and Johnson 1966: 243). They term this an 'unleashing' of the sexual drive and hypothesize that it results from a release from 'pregnancy phobia'. Indeed, they state that, other than lack of an appropriate partner:

> There is no reason why the milestone of the menopause should be expected to blunt the human female's sexual capacity, performance or drive. The healthy aging woman normally has sex drives that demand resolution ... In short, there is no time limit drawn by the advancing years to female sexuality.
>
> (Masters and Johnson 1966: 246/7)

This notion of a female sex drive which must be satisfied is further evident in their discussions about the sad fate of the 'steady legion' of older women who spend their last years without a marital partner:

> Many members of this group demonstrate their basic insecurity by casting themselves unreservedly into their religion, the business world, volunteer social work, or overzealous mothering of their maturing children or grandchildren. Deprived of normal sexual outlets, they exhaust themselves physically in conscious or unconscious efforts to dissipate their accumulated and frequently unrecognised sexual tensions.
>
> (1966: 246)

Moreover, these women are also considered to be suffering from 'coital deprivation' (1966: 241), which will hinder their chances of 'accommodating the penis' (1966: 241) in the future if a suitable partner does come along (there is little acknowledgement that this future partner could be female).

For older men, increases in erectile dysfunction and decreases in sexual desire are seen to limit opportunities for sexual intercourse. In particular, Masters and Johnson felt that fear of failure in achieving an erection was crucial to understanding why older men may choose not to have intercourse, claiming that 'many males withdraw voluntarily from any coital activity rather than face the ego-shattering experience of repeated episodes of sexual inadequacy' (1966: 270). They felt that not having intercourse or other forms of sexual 'stimulation' could cause an older man to lose 'his responsiveness' (1966: 270) or turn to 'younger female partner for sexual stimulation' (the implication being older women are not sufficiently stimulating). However, in conclusion, it is noted that the male's capacity for sexual performance may frequently 'extend to and beyond the 80-year age level' (1966: 270), depending, in part, on the availability of a compliant and understanding female partner.

Overall, it is thereby apparent that some of the key features of the 'sexy oldie' stereotype discussed in the previous chapter are evident in Masters and

Johnson's work. For example, the 'use it or lose it' model of later life sex remains a feature of contemporary writing about sexuality and ageing (Vincent 2002). Moreover, the belief that sexual fulfilment is desirable, healthy and perhaps even necessary for older people (and older women in particular) is highly evident in their research and continues to inform contemporary attitudes towards sexuality and ageing.

The Duke study (1969–81)

It has been claimed that the most comprehensive study exploring later life sexuality (Diokono et al. 1990) was undertaken by researchers working at the Duke University Center for the Study of Aging. The research was set up in 1954 to quantify levels of sexual activity and interest in later life (Verwoerdt et al. 1969), based on a sample of 254 men and women aged between 60 and 94 years at baseline. Participants were interviewed between 1955 and 1957 (study I), 1959 and 1961 (study II) and 1959 to 1961 (study III). A longitudinal analysis of data from all research stages concluded that engaging in sexual intercourse after the age of 60 is associated with being married, being in good general health, and being sexually active and interested earlier in the lifecourse. In addition, very different patterns of sexual behaviour were reported by men and women, with 'the intensity, presence, or absence of sexual interest and activity among elderly women ... primarily [reflecting] ... the availability of a socially sanctioned, sexually capable partner' (Verwoerdt et al. 1969: 1262). The authors conclude that over time sexual interest remains fairly stable, but sexual activity (defined as sexual intercourse) declines. Reasons for this discrepancy were not fully examined, but have been attributed to worsening general health, psychological factors, and a dearth of suitable partners (Barrow 1992).

The researchers involved in this project initiated a second longitudinal study, which aimed to clarify some of the findings reported above (Pfeiffer et al. 1972). Data were collected from 502 individuals aged 46 to 71 years in the first study of this scale to attempt to generate a random sample (although participants were recruited from health insurance lists and, as such, obviously not fully representative of the general population). Notable findings from this study again included an identified gender discrepancy in levels of sexual interest and sexual intercourse for all age groups surveyed. Indeed, where sexual intercourse between married partners had ceased (for 12 per cent of men and 44 per cent of women), this was most frequently attributed to the man, even when death of a spouse and separation from a spouse were excluded from the analyses (George and Weiler 1981). The authors concluded that this finding confirms their earlier study which showed that, for older people involved in a married relationship, it is typically the man who is responsible for cessation of sexual intercourse. However, they do not consider the implications this finding has for the differing nature of sexual experience in later life and, in particular, the fact that it indicates that older men and women are likely to be having sexual intercourse for very different reasons.

These data were further re-analysed by George and Weiler (1981), who studied both aggregate and intra-individual levels of sexual activity within this sample group, concluding that levels of sexual intercourse among older people do not decline to the extent that was previously believed. Rather, the identification of cohort differences in sexual interest and activity led the authors to conclude that these may be more pronounced than ageing effects *per se*. However, again, no attempt was made to discuss these findings within a wider socio-cultural and historical context.

Persson (1980)

Persson (1980) reports that, among 166 men and 266 women aged 70 living in Gothenburg, Sweden, 46 per cent of men and 16 per cent of women reported current sexual intercourse. Questions were not included about masturbation as this issue was considered 'too provocative' (1980: 335). Associations were identified for men between current sexual intercourse and better sleep, better mental health and a more positive attitude towards sex in later life. For women, current sexual intercourse was found to be associated with having a comparatively young husband, low levels of anxiety, better mental health, satisfaction with marriage, positive experience of sexual intercourse and a positive attitude towards sex in later life.

The Starr–Weiner report (1982)

Starr and Weiner instigated their questionnaire survey of 800 people over 60 in order to allow older people to 'report the inner experience of sex, as well as [sexual] behavior' (1982: 4). Indeed, they wanted to 'go beyond' the Kinsey model of quantifying frequency of sexual interest and sexual intercourse adopted to date. They recognized that 'frequency of orgasm or ejaculation is not the ultimate measure of good sex' (1982: 4) and gave a lot of space in their questionnaire for free text answers. Their participants were recruited from 'senior centers' across the United States. Interestingly, they give as their purpose 'finding the truth' (1982: 4) and stated that they 'avoided giving information that might serve as cues for responding to our questions' (1982: 26) in their recruitment presentations at each of the centres. However, they also say that the presentation 'stress[ed] the *need* for intimacy and sexuality in the later years' (1982: 26, emphasis added).

The authors reported that 97 per cent of their participants liked sex, 75 per cent felt that sex was the same or better than when they were younger and that 80 per cent were 'currently sexually active' (implied to mean engaging in sexual intercourse, although this was not stated explicitly in the questionnaire). On average, they found that those aged 60–69 reported being sexually active 1.5 times a week, those aged 70–79, 1.4 times a week and those over 80, 1.2 times a week. However, these findings need to be interpreted within the context of the very low overall response rate achieved (14 per cent). Moreover, an almost crusading attitude towards sexuality and ageing was adopted, which is well exemplified by their claim that such a 'high response rate told us that the questions we asked were tapping into a vital and hidden part of their lives' (1982: 25). There is also little recognition that their sample is likely to be highly self-selected.

While these findings were important in dispelling the stereotype that older people did not have sex, it can also be argued that the way in which they were used to promote later life sexuality fed into a growing set of attitudes about ageing and sex which ultimately disadvantaged many older people. Indeed, the negative aspects of the 'sexy oldie' myth are very evident in this work and, in particular, in the beliefs expressed that older people who were not sexually active were missing out and, as such, would benefit from receiving sex education from younger people. For example, the authors claim that while some older participants in the survey reported that:

> their lives – and particularly their sex lives – were opening up to new and exciting possibilities ..., unfortunately, this wasn't true for all the elderly we encountered. Some, who had cast themselves in society's mold of the older person, were living in a wasteland that senselessly denied them pleasure and fulfilment. And it was they, we felt, who could perhaps most benefit from what we were learning.
>
> (Starr and Weiner 1982: 7)

Brecher (1984)

The next large-scale study to be published was again initiated within the USA, and was considered to involve the largest sample ever assembled for a later life sexuality study to this date (Brecher 1984). Participants were subscribers to the Consumers Union publication who responded to an advertisement for volunteers to be involved in a later life sexuality study. Just under half (41.6 per cent) of individuals who responded to the advertisement returned questionnaires of a suitable standard for analysis. The final sample included 4246 men and women aged 50–93 years who completed self-administered questionnaires which explored a more diverse range of relationship patterns than previous studies, including marital, non-marital, extra-marital and post-marital sexual partnerships. Various behaviours, attitudes and beliefs were examined, and pertinent data elicited relating to sexual partnerships among divorced and widowed individuals. The following findings were among those reported: (1) sex was rated as more important for men than women within marriage; (2) unmarried men and women who were sexually active after the age of 50 reported greater life satisfaction than those who were not sexually active; (3) more men than women had been involved in a same-sex relationship after age 50; (4) while fewer men and women were sexually active (including engaging in sexual intercourse) in their eighties than in younger age groupings studied, a significant proportion were sexually active (40 per cent of women and 60 per cent of men aged 80 years and older in this sample); and (5) men were more likely than women to have extra-marital relationships. Overall, Brecher (1984: 17) states: 'The panorama of love, sex and aging here presented is far richer and more diverse than the stereotype of life after 50, or than the view presented by earlier studies of aging.' However, it is important to remember that these findings were derived from a convenience sample of volunteers and the extent to which they can be generalized to the general population as a whole is unclear.

Diokono, Brown and Herzog (1990)

This reliance upon convenience samples was recognized by Diokono, Brown and Herzog (1990), who initiated a community-based study involving randomly selected households in Michigan, USA. The final sample included 1956 participants aged 60 years or older, who were interviewed as part of a clinical evaluation of ageing which included items on sexuality. The authors estimated that approximately 73 per cent of married men and 56 per cent of married women were currently 'sexually active' (the term is not defined). These figures dropped to 31 per cent of unmarried men and only 5 per cent of unmarried women. Factors associated with being sexually active included being male, being married, not having health problems and drinking coffee regularly. The authors conclude that the study confirms earlier findings that sexual activity depends largely upon marital status and that sexual activity declines with age.

Marsiglio and Donnelly (1991)

The authors present findings from a survey conducted as part of the US National Survey of Families and Households, which asked 807 married people over 60 years: 'About how often did you and your husband/wife have sex in the past month?' Approximately 34 per cent of the sample did not answer this question and, of those that did, 53 per cent reported that they had sex with their spouse during the past month. Factors predicting having sex during the past month were age, respondent's sense of self-worth and spouse's (but not respondent's) health status. There was no recognition that respondents may have been having sex with someone other than their spouse.

Bullard-Poe, Powell and Mulligan (1994)

This study represents a departure from the work undertaken to date as it focused upon 'social and sexual intimacy' among older people living in nursing and residential care. Forty-five male residents aged 44–99 years rated social intimacy as the most important form of intimacy and sexual intimacy as the least important (although this was still rated as midway between somewhat and moderately important). In addition, strong associations were found between quality of life and non-sexual physical intimacy which they conclude shows that 'intimacy contributes to quality of life' (1994: 235). However, it is important to remember that the direction of the association between the two variables is unknown and therefore the possibility that higher quality of life scores contribute to an increased likelihood of intimacy cannot be discounted. Given the sample size as well, it seems premature for the authors to conclude that 'if intimate interactions are increased, quality of life will improve even for the institutionalized elder' (1994: 235). How this could be achieved is also not addressed.

Steinke (1994)

Knowledge and attitudes about 'sexuality in ageing' (Steinke 1994: 479) were surveyed among two samples comprising 304 people over the age of 60 living in the USA. The Aging Sexual Knowledge and Attitude Scale (ASKAS), developed by White and Catania (1982) was included, which 'assess[es] knowledge of change in sexual function and general attitudes about sexual activity with age' (Steinke 1994: 479). Two additional questions about current sexual activity were also posed: (1) 'How many times a month do you engage in sexual activity (includes fondling, intercourse and masturbation?'; and (2) 'How would you rate your present level of sexual satisfaction?' Overall response rates to the questionnaire were poor from both samples (16 per cent and 24 per cent). Key findings included that mean sexual activity for female participants was 3–4 times per month and for male participants, 5.1–5.2 times per month for the two samples, and that there was no difference between male and female participants on their 'knowledge of sexuality in ageing' (1994: 483).

Panser et al. (1995)

In this study 1993 men aged 40–79 years completed questionnaires asking about five 'sexual parameters' as part of a survey of urinary symptoms and health status. Overall, 13 per cent of participants were 'very satisfied' with their level of sexual activity, although the proportion of men reporting 'extreme dissatisfaction' increased with age. Sexual satisfaction and sexual drive were reported to decrease with increasing age, while concerns about sexual function were highest among the oldest participants. However, the authors recognize that their initial response rate was low (55 per cent) and that men with urological symptoms were likely to have been over-represented within the sample.

Sex and Swedish 85-year-olds

Skoog (1996) studied sexual behaviour in a representative sample of 223 women and 98 men aged 85 years old and without dementia living in Goteborg, Sweden. Frequency of sexual intercourse and sexual feelings were found to be highly related to marital status. Overall, 13.3 per cent of men and 1 per cent of women reported currently engaging in sexual intercourse, although this rose to 22 per cent of male and 10 per cent of female participants who were married. A much higher rate of sexual interest was, however, indicated, with 37 per cent of unmarried men and 46 per cent of married men and 15 per cent of unmarried women and 24 per cent of married women stating that they had sexual 'feelings'.

Wiley and Bortz (1996)

The authors set out to address the following questions: 'Is post-reproductive sexual activity a vestigial remnant, an anomaly, or is it an integral and shaping part of the increasingly large percentage of our lives spent after 50 years of age? Can it be considered a quality-of-life issue?' (M142). They surveyed 118 older people attending an 'instructional series' they conducted on sexuality and ageing, two-thirds of whom reported a current sexual partner. Some 92 per cent of the sample said they would like to 'have sex' at least once a week, although less than half of participants stated that this was their current frequency of sexual activity. Participants were asked to recall their frequency of various sexual behaviours ten years ago and revealed that overall levels of sexual activity had declined for both men and women over this time. Regarding preferences for various sexual behaviours, intercourse and orgasm had declined in importance for the men in the sample in the past ten years, while oral sex and being 'loving and caring' had increased in importance, a finding which was related to an age-related increase in reported experiences of erectile dysfunction. Women's sexual preferences remained stable over ten years and 'loving and caring' were consistently rated highly. While 53 per cent of men under 70 stated that sex was less enjoyable than it had been ten years ago, only 43 per cent of men over 70 agreed. Seven of the nine female participants over 70 reported that they enjoyed sexual activity more now than they did ten years ago. The authors conclude that sex is a 'major' quality of life issue in later life.

Matthias et al. (1997)

A sample of 1216 individuals over the age of 70 who had initially been recruited as participants in a Medicare screening programme were asked two questions relating to sexuality (Matthias et al. 1997): (1) 'During the past month have you had sexual relationships?'; and (2) 'During the past month, how satisfied were you with your level of sexual activity or lack of sexual activity?'. Thirty per cent of the sample reported having had 'sexual relationships' within the last month, and married individuals were six times more likely than unmarried individuals to be currently sexually active. Additional predictors of being sexually active included being male, having more education, being younger and having good social networks. Using the euphemism 'sexual relationships' instead of sexual intercourse was recognized by the authors as a limitation of the study, but was used because asking directly about sexual intercourse was not felt to be appropriate with a sample of this age, although they do not explain why.

Summary: Which older people 'do it' and how often?

So we are left to reflect on what this body of work tells us about sexuality and ageing. First, it appears that older people participating in these US studies have sexual intercourse (although whether terms such as 'sex', 'sexual relations' and 'sexual activity' can really be equated with intercourse is unclear). Second, it seems that sex decreases in frequency with age (although what this means to older people is unexplored, although the assumption is that it represents a source of loss). Third, there are some older people who are more likely to be having sex than others. In particular, consistently strong predictors of being sexually active include being male, being 'young/old', being in good health, and having a living spouse. (Although how this relates to a wider socio-historical context where, for example, sex outside marriage for women has been morally condemned, is unexamined.) Finally, it tells us that some older people are willing to complete questionnaires about their sexual behaviours, but others are not. Yet, beyond this I would argue that it tells us very little about older people themselves.

However, that is not to say this work has nothing else of interest to impart. Rather, it provides important insights into the beliefs of those that conducted it, both about sexuality and about older people. Indeed, while sexuality research of this type claims to be scientific, objective and atheoretical, Tiefer (2000) identifies that it is, in fact, anything but. In particular, it naturalizes and transforms into 'fact' core beliefs about sexuality which are actually products of ideas from a particular time and a particular place.

For example, implicit in the accounts reviewed above is the assumption that biology is the bedrock of sexuality. Kinsey made this very explicit in his account of how the 'truth' about sexuality could be reached so long as researchers could master the means of collecting objective facts from their study participants. Similarly, Masters and Johnson (1966, 1970) had no qualms in selecting their sample for specific social characteristics because, aside from gender, these were seen as largely irrelevant. Their assumption was that everybody's 'biology' is the same after all. The ensuing body of work also assimilated this idea and subsequently pursued the 'truth' of sexuality by focusing upon how often people had intercourse, and, in some instances, experienced sexual desire. The larger social context became largely forgotten.

As well as telling us about the researchers inherent beliefs about sex, this review is also informative about their inherent beliefs about older people. First, there is an often implicit assumption made that older people can only be asked certain questions about sex, for example, it is not appropriate to ask about masturbation or use the term 'sexual intercourse'. In addition, with a few exceptions (notably Masters and Johnson), all use self-administered questionnaires as their data collection technique of choice. While this approach certainly reflects the sexological tradition (and much social science research more generally), its almost universal adoption in the sexuality and ageing field also provokes wider thinking. In particular, it leaves one to reflect on whether actually talking to older people about sex is seen as too prob-lematic (for both the older person and, perhaps crucially, the researcher).

The promotion of later life sexuality, which forms such a key part of the sexy oldie myth, is also highly evident in this body of work. Most authors appear to assume that older people *should* be having sex because sex is healthy and fun. Moreover, that not having sex could be a choice rather than just the result of uncontrollable events is rarely considered. In particular, older women are set up as objects of pity. Not only is their (potential) lack of a male partner seen as an impediment to enjoying the benefits of sex, but their unmet sexual desires could also have wider social implications: Masters and Johnson argue that they may exhaust themselves through (over-) involvement in the lives of their families and communities. As such, a need for 'professional' assistance to enhance later life sexuality is identified (which can fortunately be an outcome of the information gathered by the research itself).

This leads us back to a consideration of what we know about older people's beliefs and experiences about later life sexuality. Do they actually want this professional assistance? The bottom line is that this review cannot tell us. Indeed, what is most striking about research to date is that the attitudes and experiences of older people themselves are almost completely absent. However, surely capturing these attitudes and experiences must be seen as crucial to furthering understanding of sexuality and ageing? So doing requires departing from the traditional approach of exploring later life sexuality and shifting the focus away from (attempting to) quantify sexual intercourse.

The remainder of this chapter will draw together research where this is happening. First, two small-scale studies which depart from the sexological tradition are explored. Subsequently, literature relating to wider aspects of sexuality and, particularly, sexual attractiveness, will be considered. While this work has not been presented as 'sexuality' research, considering it within this context is important if we are to move from the narrow conceptualizations of sexuality adopted to date.

Van der Geest (2001): Sex and old age in rural Ghana

While the sample upon which this anthropological qualitative study was based is small (including only six older people), the insights it offers are fascinating. Sex in old age was discussed in relation to 'strength', which the author infers is a euphemism for desire. Older women in particular talked about a decline in 'strength' with ageing which made sex, a 'tiresome work' (van der Geest 2001: 1395) problematic; one older woman explained that sex was harder than breaking stones. Men reported an increase in experiences of erectile dysfunction, although desire for sex was still present. Interestingly, however, both men and women over-estimated the extent of desire for sex the other felt. Older men felt that a woman's capacity to have sex was not limited by age because 'Hers [her vagina] is a path, it always lies there. His [penis] hangs, it bends down and does not lift itself up anymore' (2001: 1387). Older women, however, reported that men experienced sexual desire for longer than women because 'some men who are rich during their old age, may go and marry a young girl. If they did not have the strength or desire, they wouldn't have done so. It never happens that an old lady marries a young man' (2001: 1389). However, these comments must be considered within a context where it was not appropriate for older women to express an interest in sex.

Sex was discussed by both men and women solely in terms of intercourse – other ways of being sexual were not mentioned. Participants acknowledged that some older people were interested in sex 'till they died' (2001: 1395), and this was accepted by the younger generation so long as the older people were married and did not discuss their continued sexual activity in public. Indeed, showing restraint in emotions generally, and in relation to sexuality specifically, was seen as appropriate for 'an elder'. As such, van der Geest concludes that 'The decline in sexual interest is as much a social and cultural as a biological phenomena' (2001: 1395).

Jones (2002): 'That's very rude, I shouldn't be telling you that'

The approach adopted by Jones (2002) similarly departs markedly from that adopted within the sexuality and ageing literature to date in using a discursive approach to explore the narratives produced when interviewing 23 women aged 61 to 90 years about 'intimate relationships'. While the use of such a euphemism could be seen as potentially problematic, part of the rationale for choosing it was not to limit discussions solely to intercourse. Moreover, it enabled participants to talk more and less explicitly about sexual relationships according to their own preference. The key disadvantage in the use of the term 'intimate relationships' instead of sex (or sexuality) within recruitment materials is acknowledged within the paper – namely that discussions may be limited to the context of relationships.

Jones defines narratives as 'neither pre-existing nor a simple reflection of experience, but to be made moment-by-moment in the interaction between parties drawing on available cultural resources' (2002: 121). As such, the focus of this paper is not so much upon what participants say about sex, but rather the ways in which they say it. Analysis was directed to identifying whether older women draw upon cultural storylines of the 'asexual older person' and/or more liberal cultural storylines promoting later life sexual activity when discussing sex. In particular, the use of counter-narratives to these cultural storylines was explored and moments in the interviews where this occurred presented and discussed. Most participants invoked the 'asexual old age' storyline (either explicitly or implicitly) and discussed their experiences as sexually active older people as a counter to this, for example: 'I've had difficulties with this relationship as one always does, you know, with new relationships ... I get fed up and I think at my age what the hell am I doing? You know shouldn't I ... just be a grandmother figure at home, you know, knitting or something' (2002: 131). However, there was also evidence of the liberal storyline being invoked and refuted, for example: 'I think probably sex, and [laugh in voice] I know this is against all *Women's Hour*[1] teaching, [voice normal again], I think sex probably does become less important' (2002: 135).

The value of this paper is in helping develop a critical theory of sexuality and ageing which goes far beyond the 'how often do they do it' sexological model which has predominated to date. The development of new approaches both to recruiting and interviewing older women about sex and, notably, much more sophisticated analytic techniques than hitherto have been adopted is also very welcome.

Sexual attractiveness, 'beauty' and body image

Given the 'double standard of ageing' (Sontag 1978), it is unsurprising that most research exploring these issues tends to be feminist in focus and relate exclusively to older women, although a small amount of literature has been published regarding body image in older men. For example, Öberg and Tornstam (1999) examined attitudes towards embodied old age among Swedish men and women aged 20–85 years. They identified an interesting 'ageist' bias in terms of rating of sexual attractiveness, with 65 per cent of older participants agreeing that 'When women/men look old, they lose their sexual attractiveness' while 65 per cent of younger participants disagreed with this statement. Slightly less positive attitudes were held in relation to women than men. The same basic pattern was found in responses to the statement 'It is appropriate for old men/women to be sexually active'. They hypothesize that this may be due to a cohort, rather than an ageing effect, reflecting the fact that younger participants have been more exposed to a consumer culture where sexualized bodies are viewed more positively. However, this argument fails to acknowledge that those sexualized bodies are invariably youthful. Another explanation the authors offer is that participants may be talking about 'other' older people, not themselves. The quantitative approach taken by the study is typical of most research undertaken regarding body image, particularly within the experimental social psychology tradition. However, this has been criticized for failing to explore the meaning and priority afforded to body image within people's lives (Tunaley 1995). This discussion will continue by exploring two studies which took an in-depth, qualitative approach to examine these issues in relation to older women.

Tunaley, Walsh and Nicolson considered the subjective meanings of body size for 12 older women aged 63 to 75 years of age, identifying that 'body size has a complex of contradictory meanings for older women, which are shaped in relation to social discourses surrounding body ideals, gender identity and constructions of age and ageing' (1999: 741). Almost all women felt they were overweight, which represented a source of dissatisfaction to them because slimness was equated with physical attractiveness. 'Looking good' was seen as important by participants and weight was a crucial aspect of this. Interestingly, married women reported that they were less concerned about whether their husbands found them sexually attractive than they had been when they were younger and more able to stand up to criticisms about their weight. In addition, there was awareness that 'life is short' and that when you are older you may as well enjoy the things you want to eat, as well as a belief that gaining weight is 'normal' in later life. Therefore, the authors conclude that while being slim (and hence sexually attractive) was certainly viewed as the ideal by their older participants, age itself was seen to facilitate a resistance to conform to this notion of female beauty. Overall, they were able to accept their bodies were not 'bad for their age' (1999: 756) and seemed more accepting of their body size than younger women. This finding contradicts a lot of the writing on ageing, femininity and body image which assumes women passively internalize the youthful, sexualized ideal without resistance.

Furman (1997) undertook a fascinating ethnographical study of beauty shop culture in the USA by exploring the experiences of older Jewish women attending Julie's International Beauty Saloon. Unsurprisingly, these were women who valued physical attractiveness – Furman notes that her question about why they were attending the beauty saloon was typically met with incredulity as if the desire to 'look good' and 'look right' (1997: 52) was self-evident. She concludes that 'looking good' was significant both for reasons of personal vanity, but also because, as a woman, participants were viewed as the object of someone else's gaze. More than this, looking good was seen as an obligation. Most women had internalized 'mainstream middle-class definitions of femininity' which they felt they had a duty to conform to. Not doing so, for example by being overweight, could provoke feelings of personal shame. Similarly, participants stated that they didn't want to 'look old' (1997: 104) and their self-evaluations of their own physical attractiveness typically referred to how they looked for their age. As part of the research, Furman took photographs of the women and some participants' reactions to these were extreme. Eighty-two-year-old 'Beatrice' for example, says: 'Oh, I think it's horrible ... I really look old. Very, very bad. I look like a witch ... I really look old, old, old here. Do I really look like that?' (1997: 107).

The majority of participants used a number of measures to make themselves look younger and, in their eyes, more sexually attractive, most notably dyeing their greying hair. Interestingly, while most participants reported they do this to stop themselves looking too old, 'Shelley' stated that she coloured her hair because her 'husband chooses me not to be gray' (1997: 111). While using hair dye was seen as acceptable and perhaps even expected, maintaining youthfulness through cosmetic surgery was seen as going too far. For some, this was due to concerns about the health consequences of surgery, others saw it as 'unnatural', while a minority of participants felt they or their husbands were too old to 'make themselves beautiful' (1997: 114). In addition, three participants talked about valuing their wrinkles which they described as 'service stripes' or 'character lines' (1997: 115).

Furman concludes that the broad picture to emerge from these accounts is 'complex and disheartening' (1997: 116).

> On the one hand, women feel pressured to look young as long as possible, for *looking* old reveals the dirty little secret that one *is* old; this is a devastating admission [because]... Looking old transgresses contemporary ideals of feminine beauty, thereby denying women one of the only forms of social power and affirmation available to them.
>
> (1997: 116)

Reviewing these two studies indicates that expressing sexuality through physical appearance remains important to older women, although meeting societal norms for beauty is considered to be increasingly difficult when you get older. While Furman (1997) felt that her participants had internalized the sexualized, youthful, slim ideal of beauty and evaluated themselves (negatively) against it, Tunaley et al. (1999) argued that women in their study expressed more complex views. Being older was seen as an aid to resisting pressure to conform to the slim ideal of feminine beauty and enable a greater focus upon their own pleasure. Moreover, physical ageing was seen as natural, something over which women had little control and hence responsibility. This viewpoint was also expressed by Furman's older beauty shop customers in their rejection of cosmetic surgery as unnatural, although it will be interesting to see whether attitudes such as these are being modified by the increasing availability and acceptability of surgery which pathologizes bodies which do not conform to societal ideals of (particularly female) beauty as sick or ill, and contributes towards dominant ideologies of ageing as a disease (Estes and Binney 1991).

Conclusion

This chapter has critically reviewed the sexuality and ageing literature and identified that, to date, most of the work has been limited in scope, focusing primarily upon identifying 'which older people do it and how often'. The quantitative coital focus of the research is typical of the sexological tradition, which it has been argued, is too narrow to enable an in-depth insight into the complexities of later life sexuality. New theoretical and methodological approaches are urgently needed if this research area is to develop and two recently published studies which depart from the traditional approach were presented as examples of how this can be achieved. It has been argued that what is essential to developing understandings of later life sexuality is capturing the voices and experiences of older people themselves. The next chapter presents findings from one of the first published UK studies that was designed to this end and explored the perceived importance of sex to quality of later life.

This chapter also highlighted the need to move away from a narrow, coital-focused understanding of sexuality in order to consider issues such as sexual attractiveness and body image. A review of this area identified that little research has considered these issues in relation to older people and, in particular, in relation to older men. The principal discussion therefore focused upon two qualitative studies looking at older women's attitudes towards beauty and body image in relation to ageing. Expressing sexuality through physical appearance was identified as remaining important to older women, although so doing was felt to be increasingly difficult with age. There is evidence from both studies that older women do value the sexualized, youthful, slim ideal of beauty and evaluate their own appearance against this. While participants in one study were very negative about their own ageing body (Furman 1997), in the other study more complex views were expressed (Tunaley et al. 1999) and ageing was seen to liberate women from focusing upon other people's expectations of their own appearance. In Part I of the book theoretical perspectives were offered regarding the relationship between ageing and femininity and the oft-quoted 'double standard' of ageing (Sontag 1978) was explored. While there was certainly empirical evidence in these two studies that older women do view ageing as compromising their attractiveness and, as a result, their femininity, it was also apparent that ageing can liberate some women from constant surveillance of their bodies and related concerns about 'how they look'. It is therefore important not to view older women (or indeed older men) as passive recipients of dominant ideals and stereotypes, but as active agents who are able to assert their own individuality and power in resisting these.

Note

[1] 'Women's Hour' is a long-running radio programme on BBC Radio 4 in the UK. It has a broadly liberal agenda and often features stories about women overcoming difficulties, experiencing previously unnoticed discrimination or undertaking unusual activities.

4

How important is sex to older people?

[M]any of the topics for which data were collected are known not to affect older people greatly.

(Johnson 1997: 23, discussing why an age limit of 59
was imposed in the first *National Survey of
Sexual Attitudes and Lifestyles*)

Despite all evidence that sexuality in all its forms is essential to health and identity ... many aged people internalize the misconception that they are asexual [and] ... their self-image and self-esteem are diminished.

(Nay 1992: 314)

Introduction

The quotations above illustrate the two competing representations of later life sexuality that are predominant within contemporary Western societies. The first reflects the idea that sex and sexuality are of no relevance to older people, an idea that leads to their continued exclusion from considerations of sexuality and sexual health research and policy on the basis of age (Johnson 1997; Johnson et al. 2001; Department of Health 2001a, 2001b). The second argues that sex and sexuality are fundamental in later life and, crucially, that if they do not acknowledge this, it is older people themselves who suffer.

What is particularly interesting when these quotations are juxtaposed is that we really do not know which, if either, bears any relation to the under-standings and experiences of older people themselves. The review presented in the previous chapter highlights that these understandings and experiences are evident only in their absence from the bulk of the sexuality and ageing literature. Evidence of sexual intercourse among older people is presented as 'proof', both that older people are sexual, and that sex is important to quality of later life (see for example, Wiley and Bortz 1996). However, this association seems highly tenuous when you consider that desire does not always precede intercourse. Similarly, people may desire intercourse, but not have a sexual partner. For older women in particular, it appears that having sex may be more about contributing to their male partner's quality of life than their own.

In order to begin to explore the complexities of later life sexuality, it is obviously fundamental to start exploring older people's beliefs about the role and value of sex in later life. In the absence of this information, any theorization about how older age determines experiences of sexuality must be viewed as problematic. This chapter gives centre stage to older people themselves by presenting findings from one of the first studies which addressed this gap in knowledge by conducting interviews to explore the importance of sex to people aged 50–92 years.

Methodological background

One of the justifications for not talking to older people about sex is that, not only is this unnecessary, but that so doing could cause offence. Indeed, not only is sexuality and sexual health research generally considered to be problematic – as Ringheim states: 'there are few social science research topics more difficult to study' (1995: 1692), but specific concerns have also been expressed about doing such work with older people. Pointon, for example, considers that 'Studies of sexuality in later life tend to be methodologically difficult because of the topic's sensitivity' (1997: 6). In particular, there have been few qualitative studies undertaken, probably because face-to-face interviewing is seen as 'threatening' in sexual health research (Catania et al. 1986: 71) and having greater potential to upset older people.

However, the extent to which these concerns are the manifestations of younger people's concerns regarding talking about sex with older people must be considered. Research conducted with UK GPs and practice nurses, which will be presented in Chapter 8, indicates that while 'causing offence' represents a key barrier for professionals to raising sexual issues with older people, few participants could recount an occasion when this had occurred. In addition, North American research confirms that older people view sex as something that can, and should, be discussed within an appropriate context (Loehr et al. 1997). Within the UK, the extent to which these perceived barriers to conducting qualitative research on sexually related issues with older people hold true is unclear, as very few studies have adopted this approach. Indeed, the study presented in this chapter represents one of the first attempts to collect qualitative data within the UK about sexually related issues with older people (see also Jones 2002; Ley et al. 2002).

Study design

The aim of the study was to explore the perceived importance of sex to the quality of life of older people. The method is described in detail elsewhere

(Gott and Hinchliff 2003a). To summarize, participants comprised a random sample of patients registered at one general practice surgery in Sheffield. The practice is situated in an area of 'medium deprivation' as measured by the Townsend Deprivation Index and only 0.4 per cent of the practice catchment population comes from black and ethnic minority groups. Recruitment was stratified by gender and into three age groups (30–49, 50–69 and > 70 years). Approximately 25 per cent of those originally contacted agreed to participate in the study (this varied by age group and gender, with participation rates being lower than average among men aged 30–49 and women > 70 years). Prior to commencing the interview, participants completed the WHOQOL-100 and WHOQOL Importance Scales (Skevington 1999). These questionnaires were chosen because they are among the few quality of life instruments to include sexually related items. Semi-structured interviews were conducted at the GP surgery or the participant's own home by an experienced female researcher and lasted between one and two hours. Interviews were tape-recorded and transcribed verbatim and analysis was undertaken using the National Centre for Social Research 'framework' approach. This involves a structured process of sifting, charting and sorting material according to key issues (Ritchie and Spencer 1994). Recurring themes were identified to develop a thematic framework which was systematically applied to all transcripts. Confidentiality was assured at all times and the study had the approval of the local ethics committee.

Findings

The qualitative interview data were considered in relation to participants' responses to the WHOQOL Importance Scale Item: 'How important to you is your sex life?' Responses to this item for the 44 participants aged 50–92 who are the subject of the present discussion are set out in Figure 4.1. This shows that the majority of participants rated sex as at least 'moderately' important to them, with ten rating it as very important and four as extremely important.

The role and value of sex as expounded in participants' qualitative accounts were compared between the following groups of respondents – those who rated their sex life as 'not important' or of 'little importance', those who rated it as 'moderately important' and those who rated it as 'very' or 'extremely' important. The aim of this analysis was to identify commonalities and differences in the attitudes and experiences of participants who prioritized sex in the same way. Findings from these analyses are presented below, structured around the aforementioned response categories. Recurrent themes that linked the groups will be summarized prior to the discussion.

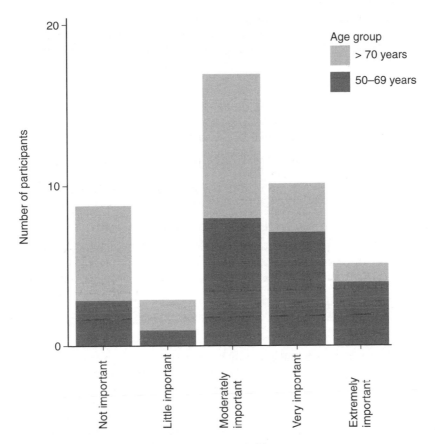

Figure 4.1 'How important to you is your sex life?'

Not important/little importance

Six women and three men aged 62–92 rated sex as 'not important' to them and one man and two women aged 56–84 rated sex as of 'little importance' to them at the present time on the WHOQOL Importance Scale. All spoke openly in the interviews about why they did not prioritize sex, as well as reflecting on what it had meant to them earlier in their lives and what it was likely to mean to them in the future. Indeed, it was their current partnership status (eight did not have a current partner, four were not having regular sex with their partner), coupled with the fact that most thought they would not be sexually active again in their lifetime, that emerged as the most significant determinants of their views towards sex. However, although this theme linked all 12 participants, individual differences did emerge when the basis for these attitudes was explored, particularly in relation to attitudes towards forming sexual partnerships in the future. For the eight participants who were widowed and divorced (and did not have a sexual partner), recurrent themes included 'not wanting anyone else', 'finding the one person' and 'running out of luck'. For the two men and two women who did have a partner (all were married) with whom they were not sexually active, physical and psychological barriers to having sex with this partner were central.

'Not wanting' anyone else

For four women who had been widowed in their sixties and seventies and not formed new partnerships following this, sex no longer assumed any particular importance because they 'didn't want' anyone else.

> Int: So, when you were with your husband, would you say that a sexual relationship was important?
> P: Oh, it was, yes, but I don't think I would want anybody else.,
>
> (widow, aged 77)

Their age was not seen as a barrier to remaining sexually active:

> I know for a fact if [husband] was here we would still be having sex 'cos he was only three years older than me and we would still be having sex. I can't see why there should be a sudden stop, you know, like I say, you get to 75 and that's it, because I mean it's just a natural thing when you love somebody isn't it.
>
> (widow, aged 76)

Not wanting to form a new sexual relationship was partly attributed to their satisfaction with their marital relationships. All reported having very good marital relationships, both emotionally and sexually, leading one woman to comment that it would not be 'fair' to form a new partnership because 'I'd always be comparing' (widow, aged 76). For two of these participants, an additional factor was the fact that they lost interest in sex when their husbands died ('You see the sexual desire does die perhaps for people like myself because, you see, I could never see myself in a relationship with another man', widow, aged 78).

However, the remaining two women did not report this and, indeed, talked about 'missing' sex. This 70-year-old woman talked about how she had had to come to terms with this prior to her husband's death, when he had developed erectile dysfunction as a side-effect of the health problems he was experiencing:

> P: I always enjoyed it (sex) (laughs), whenever.
> Int: So it was important and it gradually declines in importance?
> P: Well, it had to in my case, you take a person for better or worse. You don't say because they can't perform, that's it, you know, after all them years, so you take what's dished out to you.
>
> (widow, aged 70)

However, both these women felt that they had gradually lost interest in sex since they had been widowed and that they had now adapted to it not being part of their lives. One woman talked about how being older facilitated this adaptation:

P: For about two years it was hardly any sex at all because he wasn't well enough and then after he had his operation for the cancer, he never felt well enough, so actually, he's been gone about 11 years, it's about 13 years since I had any sex, so it's not even part of my life any more, if I speak the honest truth, I am not even interested, I got no urges, no nothing. Then again, when you get to 76, it's not the most important thing, is it?

Int: Yes.

P: It's a thing that's never bothered me, it's never, as I say, it was good when [name of husband] was here, it was a good sex life that we had before he was poorly, but apart from that I've, erm, you know, you get people who say 'oh, I fancy him', I never fancy anybody.

(widow, aged 76)

'Your luck runs out'

Interestingly, 'not wanting' anyone else was not a key consideration for the two widowers in the sample who rated sex as 'not important' or of 'little importance' to them at the present time. Indeed, one had been widowed twice and the other three times and both discussed the importance sex had assumed for them in the past, as well as the possibility of forming a new sexual relationship in the future. The key barriers to them doing this were physical – both were experiencing health problems and one spoke of his reduced libido and erectile dysfunction which he attributed to not having a current sexual partner:

P: Certainly, while ever the person has the ability to perform sex I think it's a wonderful thing. As I say, there comes a time when it just can't happen and when that happens, well, that's the end of the road unfortunately.

Int: Do you think it's just related to ageing?

P: No, I shouldn't really say so, I think when a man hasn't got a woman and he's sleeping by himself and he doesn't come in actual contact with a woman's body, you lose, to a certain extent, sexual feeling.

Int: Yes.

P: And I suppose, then, something just dies away, it just vanishes, cause you haven't got a sexual partner. Your luck runs out (laughs).

(three times widowed man, aged 92)

However, for the other widower, who rated sex as of 'little importance', age was seen as a significant influence upon his current attitude towards sex.

Around my age group I don't think it's essential really, we've been through the various stages of life and we are mellowing off. In my case it doesn't worry me in the least, on the other hand I could meet a lady tomorrow and I could marry her, I don't know, it could happen quite easily, couldn't it?

(widower, aged 80)

He added that if he did get married 'there's no doubt we'd have sex'.

'Our relationship has come to a standstill'

The idea that 'luck was running out' was also mentioned by an older married man, who explained that he was not having sex with his wife because of her long-term health problems. Although sex had played an important part in their relationship in the past he thought they would not be able to have sex again. He explained how they both felt about this:

> It hasn't upset us, we've accepted it, I mean, we had to accept it. I suppose you could do something about it, but if it causes pain to one partner in particular, then it's not satisfactory.
>
> (married man, aged 77)

The idea that being older helped when sex is no longer possible was again mentioned:

> I suppose we've reached the age where it wasn't quite as vital as it would have been in our late 20s, 30s or even 40s. When you're 60-odd you can accept it better, nor do you feel as frustrated. I'm not saying you don't feel frustrated a little bit, but you can deal with it, whereas when you're younger, it's more important. You might think of looking elsewhere (laughs).
>
> (married man, aged 77)

For an 84-year-old married woman, her partner's health problems had again led her to place a lower priority upon sex – she now rated it as of 'little importance', noting that 'we have nearly got past sex'. The notion that experiencing such problems makes it necessary for sex to assume lower priority was again discussed: 'It's just when you're not well, things change, don't they?' (married woman, aged 84).

The two remaining individuals who rated sex as 'not important' or of 'little' importance again reported barriers to remaining sexually active. However these barriers were not physical, but psychological. For one man, as well as having little confidence in his ability to satisfy his wife sexually ('I'm not the world's greatest performer': married man, aged 69), he also felt that she was not interested in sex. He explained that he would have liked to have sex, but was anxious to stress that this was not to ensure his own sexual gratification:

> I mean if my wife were ... if she were sexually interested and I would also, I would gain satisfaction, not sexual satisfaction, personal satisfaction in performing the sex act with her.
>
> (married man, aged 69)

The sexual side of a relationship 'coming to a standstill' was also an issue for a 56-year-old woman who rated sex as of 'little importance'. Although she was married, she was estranged from her husband because of past, irreconcilable marital problems and did not want to have sex with him. She also did not want to find a new sexual partner:

> I think my quality of life would be better with a sexual relationship, but I'm not a person, even though I don't get on with my husband, I couldn't go out to have sex for sex sake and just for satisfaction, I could not do

that, otherwise it would be easy, wouldn't it? I could go and have my sexual satisfaction and carry on, but I don't see it like that. I made a commitment, we are married and that's it.

(married woman, aged 56)

Finding the 'one person'

Two divorced women rated sex as 'not important' to them at the present time. Neither was sexually active (self-defined), nor thought they would be in the future. The primary reason for this was not being able to find a suitable partner, although one woman was more motivated to do this than the other:

I'm not a person that could go with anyone just as a one-night stand or if I didn't feel that way about them, I would have to be in a permanent relationship before the sexual side could kick in, you see, yes, that would be fine, that would be the answer actually, but it's finding that one person, isn't it?

(divorced woman, aged 66)

I'm not having sex and I'm fine. It doesn't bother me. If I can find someone that can look after me that's fine, but if he can't, why bother? I don't want the hassle (laughs).

(divorced woman, aged 62)

Being older was seen as reducing the likelihood of entering into a new sexual relationship ('the older you are, the harder it gets' (divorced woman, aged 66)).

Sex 'moderately' important

Fifteen participants rated sex as 'moderately' important to their quality of life. Most reflected on the reasons why sex had become less important to them, with this again mainly attributed to health problems experienced by themselves or their partners. Age *per se* was not seen as an important determinant of their current prioritization of sex, but being older, as well as being in a relationship of long duration, was again seen as an aid in coping when sex could no longer take place as frequently.

It's the 'last thing on your mind'

Three men and one woman (aged 72–76) each discussed the effect of their own, or their partner's, ill health upon the importance they attributed to sex. All considered that sex had become less important to them in light of the experience of ill health. As one man put it:

Sex is a part of life … It's a part of your living, definite. [But] nobody who feels poorly – it's going to be the last thing on their mind, sex. I mean, when I had my heart operation I felt as low as anything (laughs), you don't feel like it do you?

(married male participant, aged 76)

He also talked about how not being sexually active was expected when you were older and that 'at my age you can't grumble (laugh), you've had your time' (married male participant, aged 76). This view was reiterated elsewhere:

> You're not satisfied [with your sex life], but you have to accept the fact you're getting on and you're getting older, you know luckily if you have got a good memory, you remember when you did have a sex life (laugh). I think from an early age you realize that you're going to wear, wear out.
>
> (married male participant, aged 74)

That it was physical problems associated with ageing, rather than age *per se*, that led some participants to place a lower priority on sex than they had done when they were younger was a view expressed by all these participants. An older woman whose husband was experiencing health problems reflected upon this:

> I think the older you get and move away from what actually sex is for, it comes down to basically just enjoying yourself. Without sort of strings attached to it, it's back down to as-and-when you want, you know, and of course I suppose it dwindles, but I don't think it ever disappears. I know for myself and my husband, we have got really strong feelings and if [husband] was physically fitter, I think things wouldn't be so very different to many years ago. It's physical problems that make your sex life less really, not the actual needs and wanting, it's just whether it's physically possible, well, it is in our circumstances.
>
> (married female participant, aged 76)

She also talked about how they had adapted to this, and that physical touching remained very important to her because 'while they are touching you you're assured they're caring' (married female participant, aged 76). The potential for 'sex' to take on a wider meaning when health problems were experienced was also discussed by others among this group of participants. In particular, one man talked about this in relation to his reduced capacity to have sex due to 'his age':

> Obviously, as you get older, you act differently and you adjust to our age, but I consider that a cuddle is sex, isn't it?
>
> I mean, obviously, intercourse doesn't take place as much when you're getting older, you're not able, but the desire to love someone is there and, love, it takes a different form.
>
> (married male participant, aged 74)

'He can't make sex'

One man experiencing erectile dysfunction and three women whose partners were experiencing this, also talked about the importance of 'cuddling' and maintaining physical intimacy if it was not possible to have sexual intercourse. For one woman, this cuddling was seen as of greater importance than sex *per se* – she attributed this to her age:

My personal opinion is that as you get older, I don't think a sexual relationship as such is as important as a love and cuddle, like we do. I don't
think the sexual part is as important now that we are getting older. We
have had our sexual harassments and whatever in our younger days.

(married woman, aged 72)

However, the two other women whose partners were experiencing erectile
dysfunction did find the lack of sex frustrating:

The partner I live with he can't make sex, if you understand what I
mean? He just can't do it any more, but he's only a couple of years older
than me, but he's not interested in the sexual side at all. But I still think
a lot of him, it doesn't make me think any less of him.

(living as married woman, aged 52)

I would like sex, obviously, but it's just not there, I don't go anywhere
else for it (laughs). Sometimes you get frustrated and flare up, but then
you're all right again.

(living as married woman, aged 52)

Personally speaking, I think I could be aroused if I had a toy boy
(laughs), but of course, you know, my husband hasn't been interested in
sex for a few years now, but I think I could be capable of a relationship
which rather surprises me actually. I thought it would fade away all
together, but if Joan Collins can do it!

(married woman, aged 71)

'She's lost interest'

The impact of a partner's lack of interest, or lack of ability, to have sex on the
individual prioritization of sex was also mentioned by three married men in
their fifties whose wives were currently experiencing menopause and/or had
had a hysterectomy. For two men, being older was again seen as facilitative
of coping with a reduced frequency of sex. For one, the issue of reduced
desire for sex as you get older was seen as a key factor: 'Your sexual urge
diminishes once you get older. You can go to bed and think I would rather
have a good night's sleep' (laughs). (married man, aged 51).

However, for the other, age was seen as bringing 'maturity' to cope with
problems such as these:

It's obviously been a difficult time for her and it obviously puts that stress
on the sexual side of the relationship as well, but I think I am old enough
and mature enough to appreciate those sort of problems and bear with
it. I'm not saying that it doesn't, at times, it isn't frustrating, I think you
just accept it more.

(married man, aged 55)

Indeed, he disagreed with the idea that sex assumed a lower priority as you
get older, explaining that:

I think sex is more important for older people – I think it's more important when you're getting on a bit to show that the physical attraction's
still there, despite the fact that you have been together a long time.

(married man, aged 55)

'I've done more in these last two years'

The account of one older widow who rated her sex life as 'moderately important' warrants further attention because her experiences diverge from those
of the remainder of participants in this group (as well as in all other groups).
Indeed, she was the only widowed participant to report that her sex life had
become more important to her since her spouse had died. She described her
attitude when her husband had been alive:

I suppose he [husband] thought it [sex] was a waste of time because he
knew I wasn't right bothered. Sometimes when he was trying for me he
would get fed up and tired. There must have been something but I don't
know what it was, happen we weren't made right in that region.

(widowed female participant, aged 73)

However, following his death, sex had become important to her because she
had started using a 'vibrator' as a sex aid: 'I never felt like it in all my married
life, never felt like sex, but I've done more in this last two years than all the
time I was married' (widow, aged 73). Using sex aids was also mentioned by
a married woman who found her husband's erectile dysfunction and lack of
interest in sex frustrating. She joked that she had asked her daughter to buy
her one, but was 'still waiting' before asking the interviewer: 'Have they got
any in Sheffield (shops) … where I can go and buy myself a vibrator?'
(laughs) (married woman, aged 71).

Sex 'very' or 'extremely' important

Eleven participants aged 54–79 years rated sex as 'very important' and four
aged 52–81 years as 'extremely important' to them at the present time. All
but one had a regular sexual partner and most attributed the importance they
attached to sex to the close relationship they had with their partner and the
sexual attraction they felt for them:

Very important, but there again, it's different for other people, but for me
it's [sex] very important. He's brilliant, my husband, and that's a big part
of it and if that wasn't good I don't think we would enjoy life so much.

(married woman, aged 57)

Well, we have always had a good sex life. I suppose I'm fortunate in a lot
of ways. My missus is a size 12 and she's quite attractive even though
she's 65, folks don't think she's that age and so I think that's a lot to do
with it, you know what I mean? You've got that sex appeal type of thing.

(married man, aged 65)

I've heard so many women say 'oh no, sex, we don't want that' and I've thought, that's awful, you know that really is awful (laughs). And I think why, I can't get enough (laughs), we've got a good relationship.

(married woman, aged 51)

Four participants who had recently entered into new relationships compared past partners and relationships with current ones to highlight the importance of a good relationship as providing the context for a satisfying sex life. An older divorced man, who had been in a stable relationship for the last three years, talked about how sex had become 'a prime issue' since his divorce, as compared to when he was married and sex was not important to him. Similarly, a divorced woman, who had just started a new relationship, felt that sex was very important to her at the moment because of the 'big physical attraction' between herself and her partner. She discussed the benefits of being in a sexual relationship:

I've got some lovely friends [but] ... I've still felt lonely 'cos you tend to not feel like a woman and I've not been well over the last few years and not felt right great about myself, so it is nice that someone is interested in me as a woman and I find that to be the best bit.

(divorced woman, aged 52)

Similar benefits of being in a sexual relationship were reiterated by another woman who felt that sex had become better for her as she had got older due to being 'more relaxed', not worrying about pregnancy and having more experience: 'We know what we are doing, we've had plenty of practice (laughs) and I would never have believed that it gets better as you get older, but it does' (married woman, aged 52).

Overall, therefore, sex was valued by these participants as a way of expressing love for a partner, helping maintain their relationship, as well as for giving them pleasure and improving self-confidence, including for some women, body image.

Conclusion

An exploration of the findings presented above identified the following recurrent themes as the main determinants of older people's perceptions of the value of sex in later life:

- All participants who had a current sexual partner attributed at least some importance to sex.
- Those participants who placed a lot of importance on sex discussed this within the context of their relationship as a whole; none experienced particular barriers to sex.
- The sub-set of participants (typically widowed) who did not consider sex to be of any importance to their lives neither had a current sexual partner, nor thought that they would form a new sexual relationship in their lifetime.
- Experiencing barriers to being sexually active (notably not having a partner and/or own or partner's health problems) led participants to reprioritize the value they placed on sex.

- Participants in their seventies and eigties rated sex as less important than those in their fifties and sixties, but this was not attributed to age *per se*. Rather, the prevalence of those barriers that resulted in the reprioritization of sex increased, and became more insurmountable, with age.
- Age, and being in a relationship of long duration, facilitated coping when sex became less frequent, or stopped altogether.
- A minority of participants reported that sex had become more pleasurable, and assumed greater importance for them, as they had got older.

This chapter has presented findings from a study undertaken to explore how older people value sex in later life and under what conditions sex is prioritized. This was examined by collecting both quality of life and in-depth interview data from 44 participants aged 50–92 years living in Sheffield, UK. The findings presented support several conclusions.

First, these accounts revealed that sex is seen as an important component of a close emotional relationship in later life, although no interest was expressed in sex outside this context, for example, in the form of 'one-night stands'. Indeed, for those participants who were not involved in a relationship, sex did not assume high priority; this was particularly notable for people who did not feel they would be sexually active again in their lifetime (typically due to widowhood and health problems) and could be termed 'sexually retired'.

Second, experiencing barriers to remaining sexually active, notably health problems, can lead older people to reprioritize the role of sex within their lives. Participants discussed how sex 'is the last thing on your mind' when ill health is experienced and also expressed concerns about causing pain for their partner during sexual intercourse. That this may lead people to redefine what 'sex' means to them was indicated in several interviews. Indeed, maintaining physical intimacy through cuddling and 'touching' appears central to well-being when penetrative sex is no longer possible. Whether participants were engaging in other forms of sexual activity when intercourse was no longer possible was not explored and can be seen as a limitation of the study as discussed below.

Third, age *per se* does not have a direct impact upon how sex is prioritized in later life. Rather, factors associated with being older can lead people to place a lesser importance on sex, notably widowhood and experiencing health problems (self or partner). Another perceived attribute of older age was related to coping when sex could not happen as frequently, or was not possible at all. This was explained in terms of sexual desire decreasing with age (for some male participants), the fact that not being able to have sex was easier when the relationship was of long duration, and that a reduction or cessation of sexual activity was an expected aspect of 'normal ageing' and just something that 'had to be' accepted.

These results allow a more in-depth understanding of findings reported in previous studies. For example, although research presented in the previous chapter showed that not having a sexual partner and poor health status are related to not being sexually active (for example, Diokono et al. 1990; Deacon et al. 1995; Matthias et al. 1997), these quantitative surveys could not illuminate how older people adapt and reprioritize sex when faced with such barriers.

Moreover, it seems previously to have been assumed that if older people are not sexually active, sex is not important to them. However, this study indicates that this is not necessarily the case – indeed, only when the barriers to remaining sexually active were seen as so insurmountable as to be completely prohibitive did sex assume no importance, regardless of age.

On a methodological note, the fear of causing offence should not be a barrier to conducting research on sexually related issues with older people. Indeed, many participants welcomed the opportunity to talk about sex and discuss issues they had never talked about before (some reported that they had not discussed these issues previously even with their sexual partner). The use of multiple methods also indicated that self-presentation bias does not appear to be a particular issue when attitudes towards sex are explored with older people within an interview context. Whether this would remain true if particular sexual behaviours were discussed, however, is unknown.

This study did have several limitations. First, with only one quarter of the initial sample contacted actually participating in the study, participation bias is likely. Although this does not have significant implications for the 'logical generalizability' of our findings, it must be acknowledged. Second, in terms of questioning participants about 'sex' the different meanings this term can have for people was not fully explored (although this information was volunteered in some instances). In particular, although it became apparent that some participants equated sex with penetrative sex, this was not discussed at length for fear of intrusion. However, this reflects our sensitivities and concerns and certainly does not mean that such a discussion would not be possible. Third, the 'older people' who participated in the study were drawn from a relatively large age group (from 50–92 years). This wider conception of 'older' was adopted because the term has taken on a particular meaning within sexual health research, with 'older people' typically defined as those over 50 (see, for example, Brecher 1984; Askham and Stewart 1995; Gott et al. 1998; Gott 2001). However, we acknowledge that adopting this definition in the current study did have limitations. Notably, where the attitudes and behaviours of participants in their fifties differ from those of participants in their eighties it remains unclear as to the extent to which this reflects age differences and the extent to which it reflects cohort differences. Indeed, changes in sexual mores during the latter part of the twentieth century and, in particular, the 'uncoupling of sex from marriage and reproduction' (Hawkes 1996: 105) are likely to have had a particular influence upon the sexual behaviours of those socialized during the 'swinging sixties' who are currently in their fifties and sixties. These cohort changes, which reflect understandings of sexuality as a 'historical construct' (Foucault 1979: 105), must also be acknowledged if attempts are made to extrapolate these findings to future generations of older people. Finally, our sample was exclusively heterosexual (self-defined), although this was not our intention. It is likely that to include the estimated 10 per cent of the population of a non-heterosexual orientation (Reinish and Beasley 1990), recruitment needs to be more targeted and methods such as snowball sampling employed.

To return to the two quotations presented at the beginning of this chapter, it is apparent that the accounts of these older people support neither the stereotype of an 'asexual' old age, nor the myth of the 'sexy oldie', but rather illuminate the diversity of views held about the value of sexuality in later life. This diversity is explored further in the next chapter.

Acknowledgements

This chapter is based in part on the following paper and is reproduced with permission from Elsevier: Gott, M. and Hinchliff, S. (2003) How important is sex in later life? The views of older people. *Social Science and Medicine*, 56(8): 1617–28.

The study was funded by an unrestricted educational grant from Pfizer Ltd. However, the study protocol and all publications arising from it are *solely* the work of the authors.

I would like to thank Sharron Hinchliff for her integral role in this research and all study participants for their time.

5

Diversity and later life sexuality

The construction of an individual's sexuality takes place ... within many different arenas and contexts. Even within the same arena or context, the construction of sexuality can vary from person to person and its significance can change from one time to the next.

(Ahmadi 2003: 317)

As each individual ages so the stock of their differentness from the next person increases – the older the cohort the greater is the degree of diversity and individuality to be expected.

(Blaikie 1999: 7)

Introduction

While diversity is argued to lie at the core of gerontology (Maddox 2001), it is apparent that much research and writing in this area does not attend adequately to the heterogeneity of later life experience (Nelson and Dannefer 1992; McMullin 2000). However, where attention is devoted to difference rather than similarity, it becomes apparent that addressing diversity is crucial. Indeed, such diversity can be key to understanding individual experiences of ageing and old age, particularly where difference also represents a source of inequality.

This chapter will examine diversity in later life sexuality, focusing upon: gender; sexual orientation; partnership status; socio-economic status; living circumstances; ethnicity; and cohort (although these are obviously not the only socio-demographic lines along which differences between older people are manifested). While each of these issues is discussed separately, it is certainly not assumed that they operate in isolation and it is indeed important to bear in mind that individual experience may result from cumulative, interacting, difference. However, it is difficult to address this level of complexity in the ensuing discussions, given that most research and writing in the area of sexuality and ageing, if they have addressed diversity at all, have only done so in a token way. Therefore, while this discussion will draw findings from previous research where possible, in the absence of evidence, relevant theoretical insights will be gleaned from the wider social science literature. Finally, it will be argued that addressing diversity is crucial to understanding individual beliefs about and experiences of later life sexuality. Such insights will also help advance understandings of ageing more generally, given that sexuality is a 'peculiarly sensitive conductor of cultural influences, and hence of social and political divisions' (Weeks 1986: 11).

Gender

Gender is central to any discussion of sexuality and has therefore, inevitably, been considered in previous chapters. To recap, it was proposed that the 'double standard' of ageing (Sontag 1978) continues to sexually disenfranchise women disproportionately to men and that the physical manifestations of ageing challenge female definitions of sexual attractiveness and, ultimately, femininity itself, more so than male definitions of sexual attractiveness and masculinity. Women ultimately have more vested in bodily appearance and are expected to consume an exponentially growing mountain of 'beauty' products from a relatively young age – not to do so is considered abnormal, even deviant (Travis et al. 2000). However, this is not to suppose that men escape completely. Bodies in deep old age will never be sexual, whether male or female. Moreover, some of the traditional means by which men can appear sexually attractive, but not conform to male ideas of beauty, may further dwindle in old age. Post-retirement incomes may not be sufficient to compensate for an aged body.

In Chapter 3, the sexuality and ageing literature was explored and evidence identified that later life sexual behaviours do differ by gender. In particular, older women's (coital) sexual behaviours have been largely identified as contingent upon the availability and health of older men (Pfeiffer et al. 1972; Bretschneider and McCoy 1988; Diokono et al. 1990; Matthias et al. 1997). Indeed, frequency of sexual intercourse among the heterosexual older women participating in these research studies seemed more indicative of their partner's ability to have an erection, than the desire of the women themselves. Issues of power differential by gender therefore appear crucial to male and female later life sexual behaviours. However, research to date gives us limited information about just how gender mediates these wider aspects of sexuality. Gender is typically treated as just another 'add-on' variable, rather than a fundamental basis of stratification and, significantly, inequality.

Nevertheless, any meaningful discussion of gender within the context of sexuality must acknowledge that culturally defined notions of male and female sexual 'natures' vary markedly. Indeed, despite long-standing evidence that physiologically, sexual 'response' differs little by gender (Masters and Johnson 1966), male and female sexual natures are commonly popularized as biologically fixed and largely oppositional, with male sexuality conceptualized as active and powerful, and female sexuality by contrast as passive and nurturing. As such, 'genital and reproductive distinctions between biological men and biological women have been read not only as a necessary but also as a sufficient explanation for different sexual needs and desires' (Weeks 1986: 45). These both reflect, and reinforce, wider cultural understandings of masculinity and femininity and are known to determine how people conceptualize the 'difference' between male and female sexual behaviours (Nicolson and Burr 2003).

Such understandings about gendered sexualities have also been found to underpin the attitudes of older people themselves. Participants in the study reported in Chapter 4, for example, believed that male and female sexual 'natures' are very different. For example, men were seen to have little control over their 'animalistic' sexual desires: 'Basically, when you look at animals, a stallion will jump a 4-foot fence to get to a mare, even if he kills himself doing it, he's going to do it and we are only the same' (married man, aged 79).

By contrast, both male and female participants used more passive language to describe female sexuality and women tended to talk about sex as something done to them, rather than something they did. As one woman stated: 'Personally speaking I think I could be sexually aroused and fulfilled if I had a toy boy (laughs)' (married woman, aged 71).

The premise of this book has obviously been very different. Sexuality, frequently described as 'the most natural thing about us', is not understood as natural in any way, but rather socially constructed in complex ways. It is argued that, although biology may provide the potential for gender differences in sexual understanding and expression, how and why men and women are sexually active with whom, when, where and how are largely socially determined (Foucault 1979). From this perspective, the key to understanding how gender mediates the influence of ageing upon later life sexuality lies not in biology, but in exploring the sexual attitudes and behaviours of older women and men within a wider socio-cultural and historical context.

Recent research has gone some way to address this wider context. Ley, Morley and Bramwell (2002), for example, identified through a qualitative exploration of nine older women's understandings of sexuality that these were typically located within a male frame of reference. Having a close emotional relationship with a (male) partner was also seen as key to maximizing sexual satisfaction. Men were seen as the instigators of sexual encounters and as important in determining women's self-perception of their own sexual attractiveness, a finding also reported by Furman (1997) in her anthropological study of older women attending an American beauty salon. She quotes one of her participants, 'Beatrice'. as saying: 'I look in the mirror, I don't really feel old. I know I'm older, 'cause I can see, but somehow or other, [my husband] tells me I look nice, I look young, I look pretty' (1997: 107).

Returning again to the study presented in Chapter 4, a gender difference was identified in terms of those factors determining whether participants considered themselves to be 'sexually retired'[1] or not. For older men, experiencing health problems and/or erectile dysfunction led them to feel they would not have a sexual partner again; they viewed this as their 'luck running out'. For older women, widowhood was identified as a key determinant of sex no longer assuming any importance to them – they 'didn't want anyone else'. Further analyses from this study focused specifically upon gender (Gott and Hinchliff 2003b). We found that, in this cohort of older people, gendered understandings and expressions of sexuality were significantly shaped by the historical context within which participants grew up. For example, heterosexual marriage was seen by most participants to be the only appropriate context for sex, particularly for women, mirroring societal views about both marriage and female sexuality in the early to mid-twentieth century. Moreover, within marriage, designated gender roles in sexual relationships were identified. Women, in particular, were viewed as having a 'duty' to provide sex for their husband. As one participant reported:

> If you have a good relationship as far as sex is concerned, then you know how to use it and ... you understand your husband and if you have similar needs, or if you don't even have similar needs, you try as a woman, that is the way I look at it, that is the way I worked it. You try and accommodate your husband's needs and this is survival of a marriage.
>
> (widow, aged 78)

This finding resonates with the popular literature of the mid-twentieth century which was produced in response to concerns about falling birth rates and rising divorce rates. It promoted the idea that a wife's responsibility was 'not only [to] be the provider of food and home comforts but of sexual pleasure as well. Failure to do this meant at least tacit encouragement for extramarital infidelity by the man' (Hawkes 1996: 98), a belief that was certainly expressed by both men and women interviewed. However, participants also felt that ageing reduced the need for the woman to provide sex as part of her wifely duties – this was partly because the male sexual urge was seen to decline with age, but perhaps additionally because older women may challenge and resist socialized gender roles within marriage that were barely questioned when they were younger (McDaniel 1988), including the traditional female role as provider of sexual pleasure. As one participant reported:

> After 45 you do it, you don't worry anyway [about pregnancy], but you do it because you really love each other, sometimes I think when you're younger you feel it's your duty to do it.
>
> (widow, aged 76)

The notion of sexual liberation through ageing for women is also evident in this account and has been expounded elsewhere in the literature. Gannon (1999), for example, identifies that ageing and menopause have always meant an increased freedom for women. Such 'freedom' has particular significance for women in their seventies and upwards whose early sexual experiences mostly preceded the advent of the contraceptive pill and the concomitant 'uncoupling of sex from marriage and reproduction' (Hawkes 1996: 105). Furthermore, for two older women in our study, the notion of liberation also related to the increased sexual possibilities they felt resulted from a new visibility given to female sexuality within contemporary culture and, in particular, the availability of easily accessible information about sexuality, as well as sex aids. That sexual beliefs and practices can change over time and that older people may assimilate new ideas and attitudes about sexuality are therefore evident and run contrary to the widespread belief that older people's 'conservative' sexual attitudes and practices were fixed by their era of socialization.

Gendered beliefs about sex were seen to influence attitudes to remarriage, with the male participants stating that a desire to resume a sexual relationship played a key role in their decisions to remarry. Indeed, the central reason given by a widower of 92 as to why he was not looking to remarry was his loss of libido: 'I only wish I was still (sexually) active, I would be looking for another wife.' However, none of the widowed female participants discussed wanting a sexual relationship with anyone else: 'I could not envisage myself, the intimacy of married life, one would have to get used to another person and I personally could not' (widow, aged 78). A similar gender difference in attitudes towards sex and remarriage following widowhood has been reported elsewhere. Davidson (2000), for example found that 'not wanting sex' was key to decisions not to remarry among some older widows she interviewed, but no older widowers. Moreover, for some widows, sex was seen as one of the chores that, along with cooking and cleaning, they had been freed from through widowhood (again supporting this view of sex as a female 'duty').

Other authors have argued that another consideration regarding later life remarriage is the lack of available new partners for older women as compared with older men due to gender differences in longevity. Brogan (1996), for example, argues that there are three times as many widows as there are widowers, making it highly unlikely that older women will be able to find another husband. While there is obviously some truth in this argument, the danger is that it obscures the fact that many older women do not have a sexual partner out of choice, not because of a quirk of demography.

A further issue relevant to this discussion is the role that gender may play in mediating the influence of ageing upon individual identity, as well as gendered sexual relationships. Person (1980: 619), for example, argues that 'in men, gender appears to "lean" on sexuality ... the need for sexual performance is so great ... In women, gender identity and self-worth can be consolidated by other means.' His position is consistent with gendered attitudes to remarriage and sex following widowhood in the study, as it indicates that remarrying and resuming a sexual relationship following widowhood may be important for older men as a means of asserting their masculine identity, as well as conforming to dominant ideas about an active male sexuality which requires sexual outlets. The need to assert masculinity may be particularly important within a context where physical failings often associated with ageing could already represent a challenge to inherent male identity (although in Chapter 7 it is argued that older age can help reduce the psychological impact of sexual problems such as erectile dysfunction). For women, it is likely that ageing will represent a challenge to femininity as a result of changes in physical appearance rather than alterations in sexual function, although little information from older women themselves is available on this issue.

To conclude this section, it is obvious that the impact of ageing upon understandings and experiences of sexuality differs markedly between women and men. Presented above are only a few examples of the ways in which this can occur. It has been argued that exploring gender differences involves going beyond taken-for-granted notions about male and female sexualities and considering how these are positioned within contemporary society. Addressing this wider socio-cultural and historical context is essential to accessing and understanding the individual experiences of older women and older men.

Sexual orientation

The vast majority of the sexuality and ageing literature takes for granted that older people are heterosexual and makes no effort to explore the attitudes and experiences of those who are not. Indeed, very little has been written about how sexuality is understood and expressed in later life among gay, lesbian and bisexual older people. This is despite estimates that approximately 10 per cent of the general population is non-heterosexual (Reinish and Beasley 1990), indicating that there are potentially 1.9 million non-heterosexual individuals in the UK aged over 50 years (OPCS 2001). However, these people remain invisible within mainstream practice, policy and research.

The need to explore the attitudes and experiences of older non-heterosexual people living in the UK was highlighted by a recent study which explored the social implications of non-heterosexual ageing (Heaphy et al. 2003). Key findings which will be discussed briefly here relate to: partnership status; the role of age in defining identity; and experiences of homophobia.

The authors identified that, although the 266 study participants aged 50 to over 80 valued couple relationships highly, 41 per cent of women and 65 per cent of men lived alone. Participants identified that it became harder to meet a partner with ageing and younger participants were more likely than older participants to be in a current relationship. Regarding the relationship itself, many participants (particularly women with feminist identities) stressed that same sex relationships were very emotionally fulfilling and enabled more possibility for role negotiation than opposite sex relationships. An analysis of qualitative data gathered from in-depth interviews with 20 participants indicated that men were more likely than women to draw on 'dominant (gendered/heterosexual) models in managing their relationship' although '"gender sameness" [meant] that couples must, to some degree, negotiate roles and domestic tasks' (Heaphy et al. 2003: 2).

The authors conclude that 'Diverse possibilities exist for how lesbians, gay men and bisexuals experience, approach and negotiate ageing' (2003: 1) and that meanings attached to ageing and old age are similarly fluid. That said their participants over 50 did refer to themselves as 'older', indicating the importance of age in defining identity as a lesbian or gay man. Age identity among older non-heterosexual adults has also been explored in an interesting US study (Rosenfeld 1999), which identifies this as a significant issue because of the 'rapid ongoing discursive reinvention of homosexuality' which occurred in the twentieth century (1999: 127). Crucially, a shift is argued to have occurred in societal understandings of homosexuality from source of stigma to source of status from the late 1960s onwards, partly as a result of the 1969 Stonewall rebellion. Rosenfeld identifies that, contrary to previous expectation that lesbian and gay older people exclusively adopt the 'pre-Stonewall' discourse of homosexuality as a source of stigma, both discourses of homosexuality are drawn upon to construct identity. This is explained by the fact that although all of her participants grew up within the pre-gay liberation era, a distinction could be drawn between those who identified as gay at this time, and those who did so during the period of the liberation movement. Therefore, we return to the issue of diversity, in this case diversity in experience, attitudes and behaviours within age-defined cohorts of older non-heterosexual people.

To return to Heaphy, Yip and Thompson's (2003) study, the authors report that while female participants felt that having a non-heterosexual orientation can render you less conscious of ageing, many male participants reported the reverse, referring to 'excessively youth-orientated non-heterosexual media and commercial scenes (i.e. bars and clubs)' (2003: 8). Indeed, it is often said that older gay men experience 'accelerated ageing', an issue that has been explored empirically by US studies, but with inconclusive results (Laner 1978; Friend 1980; Bennett and Thompson 1990). Turnbull (2002) notes that the marginalization of older men within the gay 'scene' is apparent in the UK gay press. She cites the recent debate in the magazine *Boyz* triggered by one contributor's comment that he didn't want to see 'disabled or old men on the scene' (cited in Turnbull 2002: 6). This comment also highlights that older gay men face more pressure to maintain a youthful physical appearance than their same-age heterosexual counterparts. Indeed, the youthful, muscular 'adonis' represents the central image to aspire to within the gay male subculture. However, by contrast, lesbian women seem, to a certain degree, to escape the age-defying culture that can be so oppressive for heterosexual women.

Another finding reported by Heaphy et al. was that most of their participants were 'confident and open' (2003: 1) about their sexual identity, although stories and concerns about homophobia were expressed. Regarding health provision, only one-third of those surveyed felt that health professionals were positive, and fewer that they were knowledgeable, about gay, lesbian and bisexual lifestyles. It was also reported that health providers not only assumed heterosexuality, but also failed to address the specific needs of older non-heterosexual adults. Findings from interviews with UK general practitioners largely support these findings, with ignorance of gay lifestyles and practices expressed by nearly one half of participants, and homophobia by a significant minority (Hinchliff et al. 2004a).

There are also anecdotal accounts of non-heterosexual residents of UK nursing and residential homes experiencing homophobia from both residents and staff (Age Concern 2002). An article in *The Guardian*, for example, cites the experience of Roger Newman, an older gay man who founded The Gay Carers' Network after his partner of 30 years, David, developed dementia and moved into a residential care home. He reports that:

All the time people wanted to know why I was looking after David and who I was, so there was always the issue of needing to come out. Eventually I got to the point where I had no choice: I had a partner who couldn't talk, who was dependent upon me and who was showing me love. So if he showed me affection in public, I had to accept it.

Newman concludes that:

The whole caring system for older people assumes heterosexuality and assumes that you are in a straight relationship, which was some- thing I found difficult to deal with. Residential homes, though, have only recently begun to consider people's sexual needs – let alone think about their sexual orientation. (Cited in Birch 2001: http://society. guardian.co.uk/societyguardian/story/0,,526672,00.html

To conclude this section, it is important to highlight the potentially positive implications of non-heterosexuality for ageing. Indeed, it has been argued that defining yourself as a gay, lesbian or bisexual person can actually promote successful ageing (Friend 1990). Kimmel (1978) proposes that the challenges of 'coming out' as a gay, lesbian or bisexual person may engender resilience, or 'crisis competence' to cope with similar challenges that may be experienced with ageing. Turnbull (2002) identifies that the gay community is often cited as a positive factor in helping older non-heterosexual people cope with potential negative effects of ageing, such as ill health or bereave- ment. However, we know little about the attitudes and experiences of older non-heterosexual people and there is a real need to explore these in detail. Indeed, it is important that the continued tendency to negate the sexuality of older people does not blind us to the fact that (non-heterosexual) orientation can be fundamental to the self-identity of many older people.

Partnership status

While it is obviously acknowledged that you do not need a partner for sexu- ality to be relevant to your life, or even to be 'sexually active' (as presumed by most later life sexuality research), older people's reported sexual behav- iours have been found to be largely dependent on being in an intimate relationship. For example, in Chapter 3, marital status was seen to be signifi- cantly associated with the likelihood of being 'sexually active' (Verwoerdt et al. 1969; Diokono et al. 1990; Matthias et al. 1997) and, in the previous chapter, was seen to underpin decisions to engage in sex in later life. Indeed, this study identified that sex was important to older participants within the context of a mutually monogamous relationship. Casual sexual relationship and 'one-night stands' were not seen as desirable, whereas sex within mar- riage was regarded as very important at any age. As one participant said:

We have been married 61 years and like everyday people, we've not always agreed on things including sex ... sex is important in marriage, you know, and I think it's important throughout marriage until the time when you reach the age where, for illness or whatever, you can't have sex.

                    (male participant, aged 86: cited Hinchcliff and Gott 2004: in press)

Furthermore, the advantages of remaining sexually active were mainly discussed in relation to the benefits this could bring to the relationship. Sex was seen to enrich marriage through promoting sharing, trust and conveying love and commitment:

It adds to the quality of your life and your relationship, besides living and working together and doing leisure activities together but that [sex] complements it. Perhaps it's just a way of sealing that relationship ... an extension of communication really in a lot of respects, instead of communicating orally, you're communicating with your bodies.

                    (male participant, aged 55: cited Hinchliff and Gott 2004: 602)

The emphasis placed on sex as a key component of marriage is unsurprising given that it is now accepted that an intimate relationship has to contain a sexual element to be 'successful'. Moreover, as Duncombe and Marsden (1966: 220) have agued, there is increasing media emphasis placed upon the 'pure relationship' (Giddens 1992: 2) as the 'ultimate source of emotional and sexual fulfilment'.

It is therefore apparent that partnership status is important to later life expressions of sexuality and an examination of available evidence regarding the current partnership status of the older UK population therefore pertinent (see Table 5.1).

Table 5.1 Marital status by gender for people aged over 50 years in 2001 (%)

	Single	*Married*	*Widowed*	*Divorced*
Men 50–59	9.62	76.25	1.80	12.30
Women 50–59	5.47	74.22	5.55	14.77
Men 60–69	7.59	78.12	5.33	8.95
Women 60–69	4.98	66.33	18.35	10.32
Men 70–79	7.37	72.39	15.45	4.79
Women 70–79	6.22	44.46	43.95	5.34
Men 80–89	6.34	57.90	33.35	2.38
Women 80–89	7.55	19.77	69.95	2.74
Men > 90	8.07	34.11	56.24	1.56
Women > 90	10.9	5.98	81.58	1.49

Source: 2001 Census: www.governmentstatistics.co.uk

The 2001 census revealed that, among both men and women aged 50–59 years, approximately three-quarters were married, with a significant proportion being divorced. A similar pattern was observed among those aged 60–69, although the percentage of married women dropped to two-thirds. This trend continued for those aged 70 and above, at which point a marked increase in the proportion of widowed individuals (particularly women) was noted. By 80 and over, widowhood becomes the norm for older women and marriage the norm for older men, reflecting women's tendency to outlive their husbands.

Focusing specifically on divorce, census statistics confirm that this is a growing phenomenon within the older population. For example, in 1950 30,870 divorces were granted, of which 14 per cent were granted for people aged 50–59 and 3 per cent for people over the age of 60. By 2001, the total number of divorces granted had risen to 143,818, of which 26 per cent were recorded for people aged 50–59 and 7 per cent for those aged 60–69. It is also interesting that later life remarriage is becoming increasingly prevalent. In 2001, over 15,000 people over the age of 50, and 1000 people over the age of 70, got married (including seven people over the age of 80 who got married for the first time).

These figures indicate that a cohort change in later life partnership status is indeed occurring, particularly in terms of increases in divorce and remarriage. This is not unexpected, given changes in the status of marriage within contemporary society and the increased acceptance of divorce for people of all ages. There is also a growing industry being built up around providing 'dating' services for older people and advice around forming new intimate relationships in later life being given by organizations such as Age Concern (http://www.ageconcern.org.uk/1054_1153.htm). In the next chapter, evidence of sexual risk-taking among older people (and older men in particular) will be presented, indicating that 'casual' sexual relationships alongside, or instead of, marriage do indeed seem to be increasing.

Socio-economic status

> The inequalities of working life get even grimmer in retirement. The top fifth of pensioner couples now have a retirement income averaging £45,000 a year, yet one quarter of all pensioners still lives below the poverty line, which for a single pensioner means £112 a week, or £5800 a year after housing costs. What is worse – and unlike children in poverty – a large group of pensioners (17%) live in permanent poverty. Four million live in the country's 88 most deprived wards; 44% live in accommodation that is not in decent repair or thermally efficient – a major contributing factor, as Help the Aged has noted, in the excess number of winter deaths of older people; with between 20,000 and 45,000 a year, Britain has the highest proportion in the EU.
>
> (Dean 2003)

It is important to remember that many older people live in extreme poverty. In these situations, Gannon argues that 'sexuality is simply irrelevant' (1999: 124). Indeed, while sexuality may be listed as a human need alongside adequate nutrition and housing (Wallace 2003), and sex and sexual needs considered a 'physiologic necessity of human beings even in late life' (Gupta 1990: 197), ultimately a hierarchy of needs must be assumed. As Gannon again points out 'There is no evidence that sex in later life, or at any time of life, is a necessity – people who do not engage in sexual activity do not become sick, nor do they die' (1999: 111). Her underlying argument is that expressing sexuality, through appearance and behaviour, is a luxury that many older people cannot afford.

The notion of sexuality as luxury is also evident elsewhere. Tellingly, Viagra was the first UK drug to have its availability on the NHS limited – erectile dysfunction was defined as a 'lifestyle' difficulty rather than a serious medical problem worthy of automatic treatment. Similarly, one of the key criticisms of the theorization of later life consumerism and the construction of later life identities, notably a youthful sexualized identity, has been that many older people cannot afford the cosmetics, the plastic surgeries or the Viagra needed to engage with this (Phillipson 2002). Constructing a later life identity through consumerism is viewed as an option only available to the wealthy minority.

While these sentiments may seem a refreshing counter to the increasing promotion of sexuality in later life, it can be argued that viewing sexuality as a luxury is overly simplistic. It is certainly true that for some older people preoccupation with nutrition and housing will take priority over concerns about sex, but it is important not to make the assumption that sexuality is of no importance in this situation. Indeed, we know very little about how older people themselves value sexuality within the context of material deprivation. Sex was seen to be valued in above discussions about partnership status because of its role in promoting a close emotional relationship. Why should this not also be the case for older people of varying economic means? Similarly, one of the factors determining older women's use of beauty products is that 'appearing nice' can enhance self-esteem (Furman 1997). While the extent and nature of beauty products available to achieve this obviously vary enormously according to socio-economic status, it seems simplistic to assume that presenting yourself as sexually attractive is only a concern to those with surplus cash. A Canadian charity, for example, when reporting on their support in providing hair cuts and beauty treatments for homeless women, notes that 'The first woman who went through the program cried and hugged the hair stylist when she saw herself in the mirror' (Tellier 2003: 7).

A further weakness in the argument that the consumerist approach to ageing is only available and therefore only relevant to a limited proportion of the older population is that availability can structure expectation. Indeed, the fact that only a small number of older people invest in cosmetic surgery to maintain a youthful ideal does not mean that this trend has no relevance to the majority of older people. Rather, the increasing availability of such surgery means that images of what it means to be a beautiful and, by extension, a successful, older person are changing. Just because the vast majority of 70-year-old women cannot afford to look like Joan Collins does not mean that they do not want to, or crucially, feel that they ought to.

Living circumstances

Where you live, as well as with whom you live in later life, are likely to be crucial to the opportunities available to you to express sexuality. The 2001 census revealed that, 4 per cent of people aged 65 and over in England and Wales were living in communal establishments, rising to 20 per cent of those aged 85 and over. Moreover, 1 per cent of men and 4 per cent of women lived with their adult children and 10 per cent of men and 5 per cent of women lived with spouse and others (National Statistics 2001). Living with other people inevitably introduces an element of surveillance into your life – privacy becomes an issue and the views of others about your own activities can become pertinent. Sexual behaviours may be particularly problematic within this context, especially given the majority's continued discomfort with older people's sexuality.

Older people living with their adult children may find their sexual behaviours constrained. Indeed, although little is known about how an older parent's sexuality is viewed in this situation, disbelief and/or discomfort may be expected. The old adage that no-one likes to think of their parents having sex has more than an element of truth in it for many people. Moreover, the situation may be especially complicated if an older parent is having a sexual relationship with someone who is not the child's other parent. However, we know little overall about how children may 'police' their older parents' sexual relationship.

The policing of sexuality becomes even more of an issue for the significant proportion of older people living in nursing and residential care settings. Although expressing sexuality, both through behaviour and appearance, has been identified as important to older people in this situation (Mulligan and Palguta 1991; Bullard-Poe et al. 1994; Spector and Fremeth 1996), opportunities to do so are often limited. In particular, ensuring privacy when living in an essentially public space may be problematic. As Archibald identifies:

> Residential homes are referred to as 'homes' yet they are open to public scrutiny and surveillance. The expression of sexuality is assumed to be a private concern yet residential homes are arenas where the private becomes public as in the case of sexuality.
>
> (1998: 99)

In her study she asked the managers of residential homes about the sexual behaviours of their residents and found that they were able to discuss issues from handholding to 'private' masturbation (1998: 97).

Indeed, although resident privacy has been identified as crucial to achieving quality institutional care for older people (Willcocks et al. 1982; Willcocks et al. 1987), it is challenging for care providers to ensure. Bland (1999) acknowledges that normal social conventions surrounding privacy may be seen as inappropriate, impracticable or even dangerous by care staff. Safeguarding welfare is often viewed as paramount, something which typically involves a large element of surveillance, invoking Goffman's (1961) notion of the 'total institution'. In this way, privacy, alongside freedom and choice, can be taken away from older residents, leading to a challenge to an individual's very personhood (Hockey and James 1993). This will have implications for sexual identity in and of itself and, particularly, infers an infantilization of older residents which will desexualize them, both in the eyes of the care staff, but also potentially in their own eyes. Indeed, US literature (which is admittedly now quite old) reveals that care staff are uncomfortable with any expression of sexuality among older residents and typically see the sexual behaviour of residents as a problem to be contained or repressed (LaTorre and Kear 1977; McCartney et al. 1987; Brown 1989).

Residents themselves can also police sexuality. As a US magazine aimed at care home managers acknowledges, residents who share a room can take exception at their room mate's sexual behaviours, not necessarily because they feel that their private space is being violated, but because they do not agree with an older and infirm person being involved in a sexual relationship (Edwards 2003). Similarly, in their multi-media project which examined sexual expression in a UK residential care home, Hubbard et al. (2003) reported an example of a resident restricting the sexual behaviour of another resident by labelling their relationship 'disgusting' and 'perverted'. Views of other residents may become particularly significant for residents who are gay, lesbian or bisexual, as discussed previously.

The situation becomes even more complex and difficult if an older resident has (or is suspected to have) dementia. When 32 care staff were asked to list the sexual behaviours of older people with dementia that they found challenging, a range of behaviours were included from 'lewd language' and undressing in public, to married couples sharing a room/showering together; any two residents of the opposite sex continually seeking each other's company; residents of the opposite sex spending too much time together if one or both were married; and residents of the opposite sex holding hands, stroking, cuddling, hugging, or kissing. Needless to say, residents of the same sex engaging in any potentially sexual behaviour, including hand holding, was also labelled as difficult (Sherman 1998).

At a more practical level, the reliance upon the residential home to provide sleeping accommodation for residents dictates whether residents have single or double beds, which can obviously impact upon sexual expression. Indeed, although there is little written about the provision of beds in institutional care for older people, it is telling that most homes overwhelmingly provide single beds, and generally reserve double beds for married couples. Moreover, little provision for privacy and the availability of a double bed is made in the common scenario where one partner moves into institutional care, but the other remains at home. However, these are issues which are usually addressed when institutional care is provided for younger and middle-aged adults. For example, the manager of a UK hospice promotes the provision of opportunities for intimacy when one partner has a life-limiting illness, noting that the hospice has a special room for this purpose which they keep like a 'honeymoon suite' (Addley 2001).

It is therefore apparent that more attention needs to be paid to ensuring that older people living in residential care are able to express their sexuality in ways that are open to all adults above the age of consent. Balancing the need for privacy with concerns about personal safety and addressing the specific concerns and difficulties that care staff often have in managing sexual expression among their older residents are crucial to achieving this. It is therefore encouraging that training packages are being put together to address issues of sexuality in institutional care provision for older people (Archibald 1998, 2002), although it is debatable how much priority such training will receive. Indeed, many gay, lesbian and bisexual people have little faith that UK residential and nursing homes will accept the sexual identity, let alone sexual expression, of older non-heterosexual adults and a number of 'gay friendly' homes have now been established (Age Concern 2002).

In concluding this section, it is worth noting that some advocates of sexual expression in nursing and residential homes have taken debates around sexuality and institutional care to new levels. For example, the world media took extreme interest when the Thorupgaarden nursing home in the Danish capital revealed that staff have been broadcasting pornography on the building's internal videochannel every Saturday night for several years, as well as 'ordering' prostitutes for residents (see, for example, Moller 2001). Staff told the Danish media that pornography is healthier, cheaper and easier to use than medicine and has similar calming effects. Moreover, they concluded that providing these services is in line with expert advice from gerontologists regarding the need to cater for older people's sexual expression in nursing and residential care. This issue of where nursing responsibilities end is discussed in more detail in Chapter 8.

Ethnicity

No research exploring the impact of ethnicity upon attitudes towards and expressions of later life sexuality could be identified in the UK and therefore this discussion is, by necessity, hypothetical and concise. It is worth pointing out, however, the importance that ethnicity, religion and geography can play in shaping ideas about sexuality. This will be briefly explored by drawing out the implications of a paper reporting sexual attitudes and behaviours of Islamic Iranian immigrants to Sweden.

Ahmadi (2003) identifies that a crucial difference between Judaeo-Christian and Islamic views about sexuality is that, in Iranian-Islamic culture, sexuality is viewed primarily in terms of pleasure, and secondarily as a means of reproduction. Indeed, many of the rewards promised to the believers of Islam are of a sensual, even sexual, nature. However, a gender difference with regards to access to these rewards is identified. Ahmadi reports that men are viewed as superior beings to women and are thereby entitled to benefit from a woman, including sexually (Koran, Companions, XXXIX: 8; Cow, II: 183–7). Within the context of an Iranian patriarchal society, 'Men are regarded as possessing the right to demand sexual pleasure from their wives whenever they feel the urge' (Ahmadi 2003: 321), a view that is not radically different to that found in Judaeo-Christian tradition (Weeks 1986). However, it does differ from more liberal views about gender equality within sexual relationships dominant in contemporary Swedish society. The immigrants that Ahmadi interviewed, therefore, discussed how they had assimilated these two sets of attitudes towards sexuality. One female participant is reported as saying that:

> After learning how the Swedish women think about their sexuality, I tried to behave differently ... I mean like Swedish women. It was not easy at the beginning but I am working on it. I don't think that I am a passive object for my partner's sexual desires any more. I have my own sexual desires and I am proud of it.
>
> (37-year-old female respondent: 323)

While this study was not conducted with older people, it has been included in this discussion for two reasons. First, it indicates that religion and other ethnic identities do influence how sexuality is perceived and ultimately expressed. Second, it also highlights that sexual attitudes and behaviours are 'malleable' and not fixed. This finding has particular resonance for older people because it is typically assumed that the often rigid moral beliefs about sexuality that were predominant during the era of their socialization will forever channel their sexual attitudes and behaviours. However, as discussed above in relation to gender, people's views about appropriate sexualities can and do change as they grow older.

Age and cohort

Finally, it is important to recognize that the term 'older people' not only encompasses all the social divisions discussed above and many more besides, but also applies to people of very different ages. Within the sexuality and ageing literature, an older person is typically defined as anyone over the age of 50. It is this broad definition that has been adopted in this book, a decision prompted by the fact that anyone over 50 (or even 40) is typically excluded from both sexuality research and wider considerations of sexuality in relation to policy and practice. However, it is certainly recognized that many differences generally exist between a person in their fifties and a person in their nineties as a result of their age. Indeed, while it is important not to equate chronological age with health, the likelihood of being widowed, experiencing physical frailty and cognitive impairment, and living in residential or nursing care does increase with age. As discussed above, all these factors impact upon attitudes towards and experiences of sexuality in later life.

A further significant difference between the 50-year-old and the 90-year-old relates to birth cohort. As noted above, the social attitudes regarding sexuality that were predominant in the early to mid-twentieth century have had a significant impact upon attitudes towards sexuality held particularly by people in their seventies and eighties, for example in relation to a wife's duty to provide sex for her husband (Gott and Hinchliff 2003b). Similarly, the 'baby boomer' cohort experienced their formative years during the 1960s, the era of (alleged) free love and the contraceptive pill (as discussed in Chapter 2). It seems evident that these early experiences will have been profound in shaping attitudes towards sexuality, although caution must be taken both in viewing sexuality as immutable and in over-emphasizing the homogeneity of these experiences upon individual beliefs and behaviours. Indeed, more exploration of this complex and fascinating issue is required.

Blaikie (1999: 8) highlights the importance of looking at time in different ways and alongside 'historical' time, which is viewed as chronological and linear (Hareven 1977), he identifies the concept of 'cultural time'. He writes that cultural time refers to 'prevalent values and attitudes reflected in changes in age-appropriate behaviours – the styles, lifestyles and hairstyles conventionally felt to match different age groups'. Moreover, he adds that 'Acceptable age norms of dress, sexuality, pastimes, and bodily appearance clearly vary according to one's location in historical time'. This concept could obviously be usefully drawn upon in future research to explore various aspects of sexuality.

Conclusion

This chapter has explored diversity and is intended to provide both a caution against assuming commonality by age, and a spur to those interested in sexuality and ageing to attend to difference in a meaningful way. Indeed, we need to learn from theoretical debates within the wider social sciences where increasingly the talk is of multiple 'sexualities' rather than a singular sexuality.

However, I do not wish to imply that age is irrelevant. As Arber, Davidson and Ginn (2003: 3) remind us, age matters: 'First, age reflects the physiological ageing process … Second, ageing is associated with various social and economic changes … Finally, chronological age defines membership of a particular birth cohort or generation.' Indeed, age can bring similarity. However, if you look hard enough, difference is never far behind.

Note

[1] Sexual retirement is defined as the belief that a person would not have another sexual relationship in their lifetime.

PART III

Sexual health, sexual problems and ageing

6

Sexual risk-taking and sexually transmitted infections in later life

Introduction

Sexual health represents a growing area of interest for researchers, practitioners and policy-makers. Indeed, while medicine has historically played an important role in shaping and even defining what we mean by sexuality (Weeks 1989), in recent years 'sexual health' has received increasing prominence, both as a reaction to the emergence of HIV/AIDS in the mid-1980s and also in response to a wider 'sexualization' (Hawkes 1996) of society whereby sexual desire and performance have come to be seen as serious public health concerns (Laumann et al. 1999). Although the dangers of over-medicalizing sexuality at the expense of the social and interpersonal dynamics of sexual relationships have been acknowledged (Hart and Wellings 2002) and, in particular, the role that economic factors play in this medicalization criticized (Tiefer 2002), the focus on 'sexual health' is certainly a trend that is set to continue. It impacts upon how people perceive and manage their own sexuality, sets a norm against which people identify 'sexual problems' and defines the health professional as the most appropriate source of help if such problems are identified.

This section of the book will examine sexual health and sexual problems in later life. In particular, the range of sexual problems that may affect older people will be explored and, crucially, where possible, their impact upon older people themselves will be discussed. The present chapter will begin by considering definitions of sexual health and continue to examine the prevalence of sexual risk-taking and sexually transmitted infections (STIs) in older age. Information (albeit limited) regarding older people's responses to STIs will also receive attention. In the next chapter sexual problems that are said to increase in prevalence with age, for example, erectile dysfunction and 'female sexual dysfunction' will be discussed. A specific focus will be placed upon exploring the experience of seeking treatment for a sexual problem in later life, setting the scene for the final chapter of the book, which will consider the views of health professionals regarding later life sexual health management.

What is 'sexual health'?

The World Health Organization defines sexual health as:

A state of physical, emotional, mental and social wellbeing related to sexuality; it is not merely the absence of disease, dysfunction or infirmity. Sexual health requires a positive and respectful approach to sexuality and sexual relationships, as well as the possibility of having pleasurable and safe sexual experiences, free of coercion, discrimination and violence. For sexual health to be attained and maintained, the sexual rights of all persons must be respected, protected and fulfilled.

(2001: http://www.who.int.org)

While holistic definitions such as this are frequently quoted in UK policy documents (see, for example, Department of Health 2001b) and are appealing because of their focus on non-medical aspects of sexuality, they are not widely applied. Indeed, in practice, it is the medical perspective that wins through, with sexual health considered only in relation to serious health problems that can be associated with sexual activity (Greenhouse 1995), in particular, STIs. The tendency to equate sexual health with STIs is highly evident in the latest national sexual health policy document to be published by the UK Department of Health, which explicitly aims to address 'the rising prevalence of STIs and HIV' (DoH 2001b: 3). This narrow understanding of 'sexual health' has also been assimilated by the general population. In a recent study we found that people of all ages tended to define sexual health almost exclusively in relation to STIs and, interestingly, this was particularly the case for older participants (Gott and Hinchliff 2002).

Such narrow, medical and STI-specific definitions of sexual health are recognized as an overly simplistic starting point from which to understand older people's experiences of sexual problems. In the next chapter the focus will be solely upon non-STI-related sexual problems within the context of ageing. This chapter will, however, take STIs as its focus, given their priority within national and international sexual health policy. Indeed, it is important to consider later life sexual risk-taking because few others have. UK sexual health policy has exclusively focused upon younger people, for example, by linking a reduction in STIs with a reduction in teenage pregnancies. Moreover, the epidemiological data upon which this policy is based only includes people under the age of 44 (Johnson et al. 2001). Educating middle-aged and older people about the risk of STIs is similarly not seen as important. A Canadian study, for example, found that Public Health Units consistently rated the oldest of six age groups (10–14; 15–19; 20–24; 25–29; 30–39; 40+) as their least important priority to receive education about healthy sexual behaviours (Sahai and Demeyere 1996). As discussed in more detail in Chapter 8, UK health professionals also rarely perceive older people to be at risk of STIs (Gott et al. 2004). The following discussion will consider whether the complete exclusion of older people from considerations about sexual risk-taking can be justified by exploring previous research.

Evidence of sexual risk-taking among older people

Sexual risk-taking basically refers to risk of exposure to a STI, which is a function of unprotected sexual intercourse with an infected individual. Precise determinants of this 'risk' have been identified as including:

> number of partners per unit of time, number and nature of sexual acts (oral, anal, vaginal sex), use of protective measures (condoms, spermicides), partner selection, probability of infection in a partner (which depends on behavior and the availability of treatment), prevalence of STD infections in the population from which partners are chosen, and health care behavior (such as early seeking of treatment, which may forestall serious disease and curtail infectiousness).
>
> (Widdus et al. 1990: 183)

Needless to say, little is known about the prevalence of sexual risk-taking among older populations, largely because an upper age limit of 44–59 years has typically been imposed in large-scale surveys of sexual behaviour, notably the *National Surveys of Sexual Attitudes and Behaviours* (Wellings et al. 1994; Johnson et al. 2001). One relevant UK survey has been undertaken (Gott 2001), which while relatively small scale, did identify some interesting trends. Among 319 people aged 50–90 who participated in an anonymous postal survey, 7 per cent were found to engage in behaviours that placed them at risk of contracting an STI. Risk-takers were typically male, aged between 50 and 60 years and married, supporting previous US research which has identified that older men are more likely to engage in risky sexual behaviours than older women (for example, Brecher 1984). Approximately one-third of this group of risk-takers had sexual health concerns, and 10 per cent had attended a GUM clinic. Interestingly, over 90 per cent felt that they had not received very much information about STIs, although only 38.1 per cent would like to receive additional information.

The only other available UK data regarding the extent of sexual risk-taking among older people are derived from the first wave *National Survey of Sexual Attitudes and Lifestyles* (Wellings et al. 1994). Although this only included people aged up to 59 years, evidence of sexual risk-taking in the oldest age cohort was revealed. Indeed, study participants aged 45–59 reported having had more than one sexual partner in the last year (men 5.4 per cent; women 1.8 per cent), rising to 13.7 per cent of men and 6.8 per cent of women in the last five years. Members of this group of older individuals with multiple sexual partners were predominantly male and unmarried, again supporting previous findings regarding the characteristics of older risk-takers. Overall, condom use was lowest in this oldest age group, with only approximately one-fifth reporting any condom use within the past year. This finding is likely to be explained by both the lower perception of risk of STIs among older people, and the fact that condoms are not used for contraceptive purposes among post-menopausal women. Unfortunately, more recent data and behaviour change over time cannot be explored because the latest *National Survey of Sexual Attitudes and Lifestyles* (Johnson et al. 2001) adopted an age cut-off of just 44 years.

As this represents the only UK research undertaken to explore later life sexual risk-taking, it is necessary to draw upon the US literature, although it is worth reiterating that cross-cultural differences do exist between the UK and the USA with regards to many aspects of sexual behaviour (Johnson et al. 1997). The bulk of this work is further derived from the HIV/AIDS literature as little generic STI research relevant to this area could be identified.

Although one of the largest US sexual behaviour studies initiated in response to the AIDS epidemic did not include individuals over 60 years of age (Laumann et al. 1994), two other national surveys of sexual behaviour focusing on sexual risk-taking behaviours had a less rigid age cut-off. The National AIDS Behavioral Study (NABS: Stall and Catania 1994), for example, included individuals aged up to 75 years, and over-sampled those over 50 years to allow more in-depth analysis of data relating to the older age group. Overall, the study involved 2673 individuals randomly selected from 48 US states and 11,429 respondents from cities with a higher than average proportion of diagnosed HIV and AIDS cases (total n = 14,102). Individuals over the age of 50 represented 22.8 per cent of total participants (n = 3219). Interviews were conducted by telephone to gather information concerning the prevalence of HIV risk factors. Risk factors were defined as: having had two or more sexual partners in the last 12 months, being a blood transfusion recipient between 1978 and 1984, being haemophiliac (unless recently tested HIV-negative) and reporting a risky sexual partner (HIV-positive, intravenous drug user in the last five years, non-monogamous, transfusion recipient or haemophiliac). The authors identified that approximately 10 per cent of the sample aged > 50 years reported at least one risk factor for HIV infection and that for approximately 5.5 per cent of nationally recruited participants of 50 years and over, and for 7.5 per cent of the high risk cities recruited participants of this age, this was a result of their sexual behaviour. In addition, at risk individuals of this age were one-sixth as likely to use condoms during sex, and one-fifth as likely to have been tested for HIV, when compared to risk-takers in their twenties.

A second national US study which warrants discussion was undertaken (Leigh et al.1993), and included a randomly selected sample aged 18 years and older (n = 2058). Data were collected by interview, apart from sexual behaviour information, which was recorded in self-administered questionnaires. Respondents over the age of 70 were the least likely group to have had sexual intercourse in the last five years, although 44.7 per cent stated that they had had sex during this period (the comparable figures for individuals aged 50–59 and 60–69 were 92.7 per cent and 74.6 per cent respectively). Approximately 10 per cent of those aged 50–59, 9 per cent of those aged 60–69 and 8 per cent of participants over 70 reported more than two partners during the past five years. Only a small minority of these individuals stated that they consistently used condoms, and this age group in general was less likely to consider that HIV/AIDS had had an impact on their sexual behaviour.

More recently, a study of risk-taking among older gay men in four US urban centres was undertaken (Dolcini et al. 2003). Within a sample of 507 gay men over the age of 50, the authors identified that sexual risk behaviours were relatively stable between the ages of 50 and 70, at which point decreases in such behaviours were identified.

These studies therefore identify that older Americans engage in sexual behaviours that place them at risk of contracting STIs, including HIV/AIDS, although few comparable data are available for the UK, largely because of the exclusion of middle-aged and older people from supposedly nationally representative samples of sexual behaviour.

Evidence of older people attending genitourinary medicine clinics

Evidence that older people attend genitourinary medicine clinics with concerns about STIs will now be explored, prior to an exploration of issues related to HIV/AIDS in later life.

UK research to date

A small number of UK studies have been undertaken exploring the characteristics of older people attending genito-urinary medicine (GUM) clinics, which are predominantly attended by individuals with STI-related concerns. The earliest studies investigated the numbers and diagnoses of male patients over 65 and female patients over 60 attending the GUM clinic at St Thomas's Hospital in London during 1980/1981 (Kohiyar 1983). The author identified that 65 older people (51 men and 14 women) attended this clinic during a one-year period, representing 0.4 per cent of total clinic attendance. The majority had self-referred to the clinic (73.3 per cent), with other sources of referral including their GP and contact slips. The ethnicity of the sample was recorded, with 80 per cent defined as Caucasian, 18.5 per cent as West Indian and 1.5 per cent Arab. However, more detailed socio-demographic data were not presented. An analysis of the sexual histories of the sample group led the author to conclude that 'these patients tend to carry their earlier sexual patterns at least into the early period of senescence' (1983: 127). Therefore, this study would appear to indicate that sexual risk-taking practices among older people reflect a continuation of patterns of behaviour established earlier in the lifecourse.

Many of the themes identified by the above study were further explored in a review of men over 60 attending a GUM clinic in Birmingham (Opaneye 1991), providing additional evidence for the existence of STIs in older men. Of the 87 patients in the sample, 67.8 per cent were Caucasian, 20.7 per cent Afro-Caribbean, and 11.5 per cent Asian. Although this would appear to be a high proportion of black and ethnic minority attenders, the extent to which this reflects the ethnic composition of younger clinic attenders, or indeed of the region as a whole, is unclear. The marital status of the sample was given as follows: 54 per cent were married, 24.1 per cent single, 10.3 per cent divorced and 6.9 per cent widowed. This appears to indicate that there is an over-representation of unmarried individuals within the sample group.

However, it is again unclear to what extent this finding is unique to this clinic, and indeed to this sample group, which excludes women. Little is known of the clinical characteristics of these older male GUM clinic attenders, although it is recorded that 18.4 per cent had previously been diagnosed with an STI. More detailed information concerning sexual histories would be needed, though, to ascertain whether these individuals are 'lifetime risk-takers' or not.

A case note review of 242 patients over the age of 60 (191 men; 51 women) attending two GUM clinics in the Trent region of England during a two-year period (1988–89) has also been reported (Rogstad and Bignell 1991). This appears to indicate that men are proportionately over-represented within the clinic when compared to women. The finding concerning the treatment pathways of older attenders supports Kohiyar (1983) who identified a high prevalence of self-referral among older GUM clinic attenders. Indeed, 73 per cent of the Trent sample self-referred to the clinic and 'their general practitioners were not aware of their concerns or referral' (Rogstad and Bignell 1991: 377). The reasons for this are unknown, as is the extent to which it reflects treatment patterns in other age groups. It was unsurprising that a large proportion of this sample reported 'risky' sexual behaviours. Approximately one-quarter of older clinic attenders (28.1 per cent) had had casual sexual relations, 2.1 per cent had paid for sex abroad and 2.5 per cent had participated in casual ano-receptive intercourse without a condom. A further 7.8 per cent of men were participating concurrently in both marital and extra-marital sexual relationships.

More detailed analyses of the characteristics of older people attending GUM clinics were undertaken as part of a three-centre study (Gott et al. 1998). This identified that, of 25,508 clinic attenders in Sheffield, Leicester and Nottingham in 1995, 4 per cent (n = 1003) were over the age of 50 (range 50–54 to 85–90 years). The age and gender distributions of the older attenders were similar among the three clinics, though local differences did emerge in sources of referral and ethnicity. Comparisons with census data for the relevant catchment areas showed that non-married individuals were significantly over-represented within the clinic samples as a whole. There was an association between age and diagnostic profile with older patients more likely to be diagnosed with non-sexually transmitted infections and infections not requiring treatment. Furthermore, proportionately smaller numbers of older people were tested for HIV, especially among male patients. The authors conclude that, if clinic attendance within this age group throughout England were consistent with these three clinics, total number of cases seen in individuals over the age of 50 would approach 16,000 for 1995.[1] In addition, when compared with younger attenders, these older patients do exhibit distinct diagnostic and demographic profiles.

The follow-up to this study gathered more detailed information from older GUM clinic attenders themselves (Gott et al. 2000). A self-administered questionnaire study linked to patient note data was undertaken within the same three GUM clinics in the Trent region. Participants comprised 224 individuals aged 50 years and older attending the three clinics during the study period. The majority of study participants were attending the clinic with a suspected STI (n = 145; 64.7 per cent) and approximately half (53.1 per cent; n = 119) were first-time GUM clinic attenders. Participants cited the suspected source of their infection as follows: 'past sexual partner' (14.5 per cent; n = 21), 'no-one in particular' (13.8 per cent; n = 20), 'long-term sexual partner' (11.7 per cent; n = 17), 'new sexual partner' (11.0 per cent; n = 16) and spouse (7.6 per cent; n = 11). However, 33.1 per cent (n = 48) stated that they did not know from whom they had contracted the infection or condition. Data available only for participants recruited from the Sheffield clinic indicated that, although the majority of participants reported having had only one sexual partner during the past 12 months, a significant minority reported considerable higher numbers of partners, including partners classed 'higher risk' for STI acquisition. These data confirm that older people in the UK engage in behaviours that place them at risk of STI acquisition and many attend GUM clinics for the first time in later life.

Further analyses from these study data focused upon the sub-sample of 121 symptomatic older patients attending with a suspected STI (Gott et al. 1999). These identified that 43.8 per cent (n = 53) of these patients waited over two weeks between symptom recognition and clinic attendance. Reasons given for delay included wanting to 'wait and see' if symptoms improved and being embarrassed or afraid to attend the clinic. Of particular significance was that comparisons with previous research (Fortenberry 1997) indicated that levels of delay behaviour reported by this older sample are higher than those exhibited by youthful populations with STI-attributed symptoms. This finding is significant given that the importance of seeking prompt medical treatment for suspected STIs is well established, with specific implications of delayed presentation including potential transmission of infection to sexual partners and the development of complicating sequelae for infected individuals (Aral and Wasserheit 1997).

HIV/AIDS and older people

Approximately 11 per cent of cases of AIDS and 7 per cent of cases of HIV in the UK have been diagnosed in individuals over the age of 50 (Table 6.1). Moreover, the total number of people over 50 infected with HIV and AIDS will be greater because these data refer only to age at diagnosis, not the current prevalence of infection by age group. Indeed, it is important to remember that the advent of anti-retroviral therapies and a concomitant shift to seeing HIV as a chronic, rather than a terminal, illness (Flowers et al. 2003), has resulted in an increasing proportion of people entering later life with HIV.

Table 6.1 UK AIDS cases and HIV infection for individuals aged 50 and over at diagnosis, by sex: to end of December 2003

Age	Male				Female			
	HIV		AIDS		HIV		AIDS	
	No.	(%)	No.	(%)	No.	(%)	No.	(%)
All ages	45,530	100	16,903	100	15,226	100	3,190	n/a
50–54	1742	4	971	6	282	2	79	2
55–59	966	2	574	3	170	1	55	2
60–64	552	1	316	2	74	0.5	36	1
65+	353	1	211	1	54	0.5	21	1
Total aged > 50 years	3613	8	2072	12	580	4	191	6

Source: Health Protection Agency (HIV/STI Department, Communicable Disease Surveillance Centre) and the Scottish Centre for infection and Environmental Health (2004)

By far the most common source of transmission for people over 50 has been through men having sex with men, which represents nearly two-thirds of male HIV infections and nearly three-quarters of male AIDS diagnoses. However, transmission through heterosexual intercourse is also relatively high; 15.5 per cent of all male cases of AIDS transmitted through heterosexual sex have been among men over the age of 50 (the comparable figure for women is 6.6 per cent). Only very small numbers of older people have been infected through intravenous drug use (Health Protection Agency (HIV/STI Department, Communicable Disease Surveillance Centre) and the Scottish Centre for Infection and Environmental Health, Unpublished Quarterly Surveillance 2004)).

In the USA, 13 per cent of AIDS diagnoses and 7 per cent of HIV diagnoses have been made in people over the age of 50 (Centers for Disease Control and Prevention 2001). While the proportion of older people with HIV/AIDS is similar within the USA and the UK, the majority of literature reviewed in this section is from the USA as only a few very small-scale studies have been undertaken within the UK.

North American literature

Studies identifying the presence of HIV in older cohorts will be examined first. Research addressing the implications of HIV within older populations for both health care professionals and older people themselves will then be discussed.

A study instigated early on in the AIDS epidemic involved analysing data routinely collected by the Center for Disease Control (CDC) with the aim of compiling a descriptive epidemiology of HIV and AIDS cases diagnosed among individuals over the age of 50 (Ship et al. 1991). Comparisons were made with individuals under the age of 50 in order to identify any age-specific trends. Approximately 10 per cent of AIDS diagnoses (n = 11,984) up to December 1989 were identified as being in individuals over the age of 50; 7.3 per cent were aged 50–59 years (n = 8480), 2.4 per cent were aged 60–69 years (n = 2741), and 0.7 per cent (n = 763) over 70. Exposure categories were distinct for older individuals, with those over 50 more likely to have acquired HIV by transfusion, or to have an indeterminable means of infection. However, the majority of cases were transmitted through men having sex with men for all ages under 70 years, although heterosexual transmission was also recognized as important. The percentage of patients diagnosed in the same month as death rose sharply by age to 37 per cent in those aged over 80 years. That older people were more likely to have an indeterminable mode of HIV transmission was attributed to reticence on the part of individuals of this age group in reporting information on sexual behaviour and intravenous drug use. This finding, coupled with the fact that there was an increase in diagnosis in the same month as death for older people, indicates a reluctance on the part of health care professionals to explore sexual histories, or to consider STI diagnoses among this age group, as will be discussed in more detail in Chapter 8.

The issue of under-diagnosis was also addressed in a study which involved testing all individuals over the age of 60 who had died in the Harlem Hospital Center, New York, for presence of the HIV antibody (El-Sadr and Gettler 1995); patients diagnosed with HIV/AIDS prior to death were excluded from the study. A significant minority of those tested (5.05 per cent; n = 13) were found to be HIV-antibody positive, although hospital personnel had not previously identified this diagnosis. Indeed, none of these individuals had been tested for HIV, despite having risk factors for the virus, including intravenous drug use. Although it is stressed that these findings cannot be extrapolated either to the general population, or to other older hospital patients, this study does confirm that health care professionals do not anticipate older people's risk of acquiring HIV/AIDS.

The characteristics of individuals over the age of 60 diagnosed with HIV or AIDS within a large urban hospital have also been described (Gordon and Thompson 1995). It was found that this group included over five times as many men as women, and that the primary risk factor for HIV/AIDS transmission was homosexual or bisexual intercourse. Furthermore, the majority of patients presenting with characteristic HIV symptoms had not been tested for HIV immediately, but had waited a median of 3.1 months (range 1–10 months) before this was suggested by their doctor.

A study of HIV prevalence and risk behaviour data among 2881 men who have sex with men (MSM) aged 50 years or older was conducted in 1997 in New York, Los Angeles, Chicago, and San Francisco and analyses were presented for the 507 participants over the age of 50 (Dolcini et al. 2003). Nineteen per cent of men in their fifties, 3 per cent of men in their sixties, but no men in their seventies were identified as HIV positive (HIV status was identified through self-report and biologic measures). The lower levels of infection among men in their sixties and seventies was attributed to high levels of AIDS mortality among older gay men prior to the availability of highly active retroviral therapy. Particularly high rates of infection were found among older black participants (30 per cent), older gay men who were injection drug users (21 per cent), moderately heavy drug users (35 per cent), and, what the authors term 'less closeted men' (21 per cent). It is concluded that 'current levels of HIV among older urban MSM in the United States are very high, particularly among those in their 50s' (Dolcini et al. 2003: S115).

The first large-scale, representative sample of older people with HIV in the USA has also been conducted recently (Zingmond et al. 2002), exploring individual circumstances at diagnosis and disease progression in a probability sample of 2864 HIV positive adults, including 286 over the age of 50. The authors identified that older people were more likely to be diagnosed with HIV when they had symptoms and that older non-White participants had a more rapid disease progression than older White participants. A key implication of this study is that it indicates that HIV infection is likely to be under-reported among older individuals, casting doubt on the accuracy of published HIV datasets. While comparable information is not available for the UK, there is no reason to suggest that late diagnosis of HIV among the older population is specific to the USA.

Nichols et al. (2002) report the findings of a survey of 172 people > 45 years living with HIV in the West Florida area, instigated due to the increasing prevalence of HIV in the older population of this area, coupled with concerns about high levels of unmet service need in this group. This included a qualitative component and was largely focused upon satisfaction with, and need for, services. Interesting findings included: (1) high levels of education in this cohort in combination with dramatically low current income levels and high rates of poverty; (2) high prevalence of historical risk events (e.g. sexual abuse) and behaviours; and (3) high rates of psychological morbidity (this sample were nearly 15 times more likely to be experiencing severe depression than the general population). Moreover, the particular stigma of being diagnosed with HIV as an older person also emerged as an interesting and important finding, as explored in more detail below.

UK literature

Very little has been written in the UK about HIV/AIDS and older adults. Only four original studies could be identified, all of which are very small-scale. Rickard (1995) described the characteristics, living situations and carer support available for a sample of six HIV positive individuals over 55 years of age. She identified that these individuals experienced a high degree of social isolation and, because of their age, did not feel comfortable using general HIV services.

Similar findings are reported in a study undertaken in collaboration with Age Concern (Youdell et al. 1995). Thirty people were interviewed, of whom five were living with HIV/AIDS, eight were partners or parents of people with HIV/AIDS and 17 were employed by statutory or voluntary services. Key recommendations include the tailoring of services more specifically to older people, the need for support for carers and the provision of a befriending scheme for older people with HIV/AIDS.

Review articles have also been provided (Marr 1994a, 1994b), drawing attention to the need for additional research in this area and Age Concern has produced a number of relevant publications (Age Concern 1995; Kaufman 1995). These include case studies taken from interviews with older people with HIV and AIDS and also specific information for people with AIDS, their carers, family and friends and health care professionals.

This brief review has identified that older people do contract HIV/AIDS, although they do not seem to be perceived as susceptible to this condition by health care professionals, an issue which will receive more attention in Chapter 8.

Educating older people about sexually transmitted infections

> Effective health education needs a two-pronged approach, aimed in a general way at *all young people*, and also at those identified at particularly 'high risk'. *Young people* have a right to sound, unbiased information that allows them to make informed choices before they have sexual intercourse.
>
> (Adler 1997: 1746: emphasis added)

As indicated in this quote, STI health promotion campaigns have almost exclusively been targeted at younger age groups (Kaufmann 1995). The literature used in such campaigns makes this explicit – while leaflets may show images of people of different ethnic backgrounds and sexual orientations, they all typically share at last one common characteristic, namely youth. This reinforces the message that STIs are not of relevance to anyone over the age of 40.

Research undertaken with older people confirms that this age group do not feel that they have received very much information about STIs, including HIV/AIDS. Indeed, in two samples of people over the age of 50, one recruited from a GUM clinic, and the other from the general population, most felt they had received 'hardly any' or 'not very much' information about this aspect of sexual health (Gott et al. 2000). Both groups had gleaned most of their knowledge about STIs from the media or television, although as would be expected, those recruited from the clinic also identified GUM health professionals as a significant information source. Approximately one-quarter of participants in both studies reported that they would like to receive more information about STIs. For the general population sample, the preferred source of this information was the media, closely followed by the GP. By contrast, the clinic sample cited GUM professionals as their favoured source of information, again closely followed by their GP.

It is therefore apparent that there is a significant need to make more information about STIs available to older people. This may not only help older people who have concerns about their own sexual health, but could also assist them in addressing the worries of friends and family members. Indeed, it is important to remember that older people often play a significant role in imparting information and knowledge to members of their family (Bullock 2001) and even their wider community. Moreover, a need for information may also relate to their more specific caring roles. While it is not known how many older people in the UK are caring for grandchildren in place of children who are seriously ill or have died from AIDS, figures from the USA indicate that many older people do fulfil this caring role (Poindexter and Linsk 1999). In Sub-Saharan Africa, where seven out of ten new cases of HIV are diagnosed (UNAIDS 2002), older people (and older women in particular) are 'key resources for combating AIDS and alleviating its impact' (deGraft et al. 2002: 2). Here, the potential benefits that educating older people about STIs and HIV/AIDS can have for the community as a whole is well recognized (deGraft et al. 2002).

To conclude this section, it is important to stress that it is certainly not being proposed that education efforts around STIs should be targeted primarily at older people. Younger people remain disproportionately at risk of STIs and education is particularly important when norms for sexual behaviour are being developed. However, it is being argued that *exclusively* targeting younger people is misguided. Not only does it impart the message that older people are in some way immune from contracting STIs which, as has been seen above, is certainly not the case, but it also fails to recognize the role older people can play in educating and caring for younger members of their family.

The experience of older people diagnosed with an STI

Unfortunately, we know very little about the impact of STI diagnoses upon older people. Most work undertaken exploring STIs in later life has focused upon establishing whether older people are at risk of, and do contract these infections. Having established that this is indeed the case, there is a need for research to become theoretically and methodologically more sophisticated in focus and address how older people themselves understand and experience STIs.

Research undertaken with younger people does indicate that contracting an STI has very particular implications within contemporary society. Most notably, such a diagnosis can lead to public disclosure of private or intimate behaviours (Gilmore and Somerville 1994) and, if those behaviours do not meet with societal approval, the illness can be stigmatized (Sontag 1991). This was highly evident at the onset of the AIDS pandemic when gay men were initially disproportionately infected and the term 'the gay plague' was bandied around. Even today there are still distinctions drawn between the 'innocent victims' of AIDS, notably haemophiliacs and children, and those who continue to be blamed for their own condition. As Weeks states:

> In the fear and loathing that AIDS evokes there is a resulting conflation between two plausible, if unproven theories – that there is an elective affinity between disease and certain sexual practices, and that certain sexual practices cause disease – and a third, that certain types of sex *are* diseases.
>
> (1985: 46)

That there continues to be real stigma attached to becoming infected with a sexually transmitted condition is confirmed by research undertaken with younger people (Holgate and Longman 1998; Duncan et al. 2001). A study exploring the impact of a diagnosis of *Chlamydia trachomatis* on women attending a GUM clinic in Glasgow (Duncan et al. 2001), for example, identified significant embarrassment and personal disgust among this patient group. One participant, reported that being diagnosed with chlamydia made her feel 'really dirty, because it's an STD [sexually transmitted disease] basically and I thought people like me don't get these kinds of things (2001: 196).

It is unsurprising that the stigma attached to contracting an STI can inhibit treatment seeking (Leenars et al. 1993; Duncan et al. 1995). A qualitative study with younger patients, for example, identified that perceptions of GUM clinics can be highly negative, as indicated by the following extract from an interview conducted with a young woman recently diagnosed with an STI:

Int: What did you think about the [GUM] clinic before you went [there]?

P: ... like seedy, seedy people and people that are – not, not prostitutes, I wouldn't go so far as to say that, but just a lot ... that sort of place, you know, like filthy men go and a lot of men sitting about.

(cited in Scoular et al. 2001: 341)

There is evidence that older people share these views about GUM clinics, and indeed may even perceive them more negatively. For example, in one of the studies discussed above, it was noted that 43.8 per cent (n = 53) of GUM clinic attenders aged > 50 years had waited over two weeks between symptom recognition and clinic attendance, a level of delay behaviour that is higher than that found among younger patients (Fortenberry 1997). Reasons given for delaying treatment seeking revealed that is due in part to being embarrassed or afraid to do so, indicating that older people do perceive a stigma attached to seeking treatment for an STI. Moreover, they may feel out of place when attending a GUM clinic given that the majority of the patients are younger and that sexual health information displayed is typically youth orientated. However, these issues have not been explored to date and require further attention.

Information gathered from older people with HIV/AIDS indicates that there is a particular stigma attached to contracting this condition. A US study exploring various implications of HIV diagnosis in later life found, for example, that being diagnosed with HIV as an older person was perceived as very difficult. The experience of 'Tony', who was newly diagnosed with HIV at the age of 70, is cited. He states that:

HIV diminished me, ... it kind of made me feel almost like a sub-species ... It was quite shattering. I just felt that, all of a sudden, I became inferior. I might have felt quite similar to that if I had been diagnosed with something else that would be considered terminal ... but I think the social implications of HIV came into it quite a bit.

(Nichols et al. 2002: 75)

A small-scale study commissioned by Age Concern reports similar findings

(Youdell et al. 1995), with service providers in particular reporting that older people with IIIV could be excluded from services because of their age. Moreover, specialist HIV voluntary services were seen to be geared to the needs of younger people and not appropriate for older people. For example, one male participant reported that he found the fact that the majority of those using the services young problematic: 'they're all so young, that put me off' (1995: 20).

Conclusion

The limitations of research undertaken to date exploring sexual risk-taking and STIs in later life have already been highlighted in the introduction and any implications drawn from this body of work must be viewed within this context. However, there are some key trends that can be identified as relevant to understandings of these issues.

1 People over 50 do engage in sexual behaviours which place them at risk of STIs and do seek treatment for, and are diagnosed with, STIs.
2 Sexual risk-takers are more likely to be male and include both married men and those without a current long-term partner.
3 The majority of older people attend a GUM clinic for the first time in later life.
4 Older people are less likely than any other age group to use condoms, probably reflecting a need not to use contraception when women are post-menopausal, but also potentially a belief that they are not at risk of STIs.
5 Approximately 7 per cent of HIV infections and 11 per cent of AIDS cases in the UK have been diagnosed in people over the age of 50. The dominant mode of transmission in this older age group is men having sex with men, although heterosexual transmission is also significant.
6 There is evidence that older people are not perceived to be at risk of STIs by health care professionals, for example, HIV/AIDS may be diagnosed late in the disease progression, or not at all.
7 STI-related health promotion is directed at youthful populations. However, there is a need to educate older people about this issue, not only because their own sexual behaviours may place them at risk of infection, but also because they can play a role in educating younger members of their family about sexual risk-taking.
8 Older people contracting STIs are likely to experience the general stigma that affects anyone who contracts a sexually acquired condition, but also may be particularly isolated and marginalized because of their age.

This chapter has identified that, contrary to popular belief, a significant minority of older people do engage in 'risky' sexual behaviours and contract STIs. Moreover, a consideration of the demographic and social changes likely to be experienced over the coming decades indicates that rates of STIs within older age groups can only be set to rise. The expectations of older people in this country are changing. Indeed, not only will demographic change ensure that there are more older people in the future than ever before, but these people are likely to be more sexually active, have more sexual partners, and be more vocal about their sexual health concerns than previous generations. However, there is little indication that national policy positions on STI-related health issues in later life will respond to these wider social and demographic shifts.

Acknowledgements

Extracts from this chapter have been published previously and are reproduced with the permission of Cambridge University Press from Gott, M. (2004) Are older people at risk of sexually transmitted infections? A new look at the evidence. Reviews in *Clinical Gerontology* (in press), copyright Cambridge University Press.

Note

[1] Estimate based on total cases seen in GUM clinics in England in 1995 and 1996 according to GUM workload statistics.

7

Sexual 'dysfunctions' and ageing

Introduction: What counts as 'sexually dysfunctional'?

> [Sexual dysfunction is] characterized by a disturbance in the processes that characterize the sexual response cycle or by pain associated with sexual intercourse.
>
> (American Psychiatric Association 1994: 493)

> What is the 'function' that 'sexual dysfunction' threatens? Quite simply, it is penile-vaginal intercourse in the marital (or at least stable heterosexual) unit. The 'function' is 'successful' intercourse, which is 'functional' for the couple, which is 'functional' for society.
>
> (Marshall 2002: 134)

The medical gold standard definition of sexual dysfunction is provided by the *Diagnostic and Statistical Manual of Disorders*, fourth edition (DSM-IV), developed by the American Psychiatric Association and revised most recently in 1994. The 'cycle' referred to in the above quotation is the 'Human Sexual Response Cycle' (HSRC) originally proposed by Masters and Johnson (1966, 1970) to describe the key sequential stages of 'normal' sexual functioning, namely sexual drive, desire, arousal and orgasm. DSM-IV splits the types of dysfunctions that can arise in this cycle for both men and women into four categories: sexual desire disorders, sexual arousal disorders, orgasmic disorders, and sexual pain disorders.

Despite underpinning most contemporary thought about what constitutes sexual normalcy, the DSM classification of sexual dysfunction has been subject to extensive critique. First, it is apparent that so-called 'normal' sexual functioning is defined as mutual orgasm following heterosexual intercourse. However, the extent to which this can be considered normal is highly debatable. For example, as noted in Chapter 2, orgasm during heterosexual intercourse is neither commonplace for women (Kinsey et al. 1953; Nicolson 1993, 1994) nor central to women's definitions of pleasurable sex (Hite 1989; Nicolson and Burr 2003). Therefore, defining 'anorgasmia' (persistent or recurrent delay in, or absence of, orgasm, following a normal sexual excitation phase: American Psychiatric Association 1994) as a sexual dysfunction appears immediately problematic. Moreover, how a 'normal' sexual excitation phase is defined remains unclear. In a similar vein, can 'hypoactive sexual desire' (persistently or recurrently deficient, or absent, sexual fantasies and desire for sexual activity: American Psychiatric Association 1994), the most prevalent sexual dysfunction identified among women, really be considered a medically diagnosable condition? In commenting on a study in which 41 per cent of women reported 'lack of interest in sex' during the last year (Mercer et al. 2003), Katz (2003) highlights that women were not asked whether this constituted a problem to them. As such, she argues that categorizing these women as dysfunctional is highly problematic given that:

> For many women, lack of interest [in sex] has more to do with the context of their lives and may in fact be protective. If a woman does not have a partner or is stressed with multiple role demands, lack of interest in sex may actually be adaptive in that she can focus on other important issues in her life.
>
> (http://bmj.bmjjournals.com/cgi/eletters/327/7412/426#36098)

Further criticisms have been levelled against the HSRC, the model underpinning definitions of sexual dysfunction. As noted briefly in Chapter 3, the 'discovery' of the Human Sexual Response Cycle (Masters and Johnson 1966, 1970) has been argued to be 'a self-fulfilling prophecy' (Tiefer 1995: 44). In particular, it has been highlighted that participants' sexual experiences had to correspond to the norms of the cycle to meet the initial recruitment criteria; in other words, they had to report having had an orgasm following (heterosexual) intercourse. Moreover, participants were also purposively selected for 'intelligence' and the final sample was overwhelmingly middle-class, white, and middle-aged. It therefore appears highly problematic to view these participants' experiences as forming the basis of a universal model of human sexual functioning.

In recent years, further challenges have been levelled at the DSM-IV, particularly in relation to debates on 'female sexual dysfunction' (as described in Chapter 2). In proposing a 'new view of women's sexual problems' (The Working Group for a New View of Women's Sexual Problems 2001: 1) the following criticisms of the DSM classification have been made (2001: 4–5). First, it is argued that it draws a false equivalency between male and female sexuality, for example, there is empirical evidence that women's sexual experiences do not neatly correspond with the HSRC, for example, many women care less about physical than subjective arousal (Hite 1989; Ellison 2000). In addition, DSM-IV erases the relational context of sexuality and ignores the fact that intimacy often lies at the root of sexual satisfaction and sexual problems (The Working Group for a New View of Women's Sexual Problems 2001); when viewing the DSM-IV classification, sexuality appears to consist solely of discrete genital functioning. Finally, the 'levelling of differences' is criticized – women (although this obviously applies equally to men) are argued to differ in their attitudes towards sexuality and in their social and cultural backgrounds, something that is not accommodated by a 'one-size-fits-all' diagnosis (Working Group 2001: 3).

It therefore becomes immediately apparent that there are real problems in accepting medical definitions of sexual dysfunction. However, this has largely been ignored in most of the wider sexuality and health literature, which has rather gone to great lengths to identify the prevalence of these dysfunctions in various populations. More worryingly still, few have acknowledged that equivalency cannot be drawn between sexual dysfunctions and sexual problems. For example, on the basis of surveys claiming that 'female sexual dysfunction' (classified as any of the four categories of dysfunction in DSM-IV as described above) affects 41–43 per cent of the female population of both the UK (Read et al. 1997; Dunn et al. 1998) and the USA (Laumann et al. 1999), it has been argued that this 'disease' represents a significant public health concern (Laumann et al. 1999). However, these surveys did not take into account whether identified dysfunctions were perceived as such by study participants. It therefore seems deeply problematic to claim that sexual dysfunctions are a public health concern, given that we do not even know the extent to which these represented a concern to the women affected. Furthermore, in relation to older people, it is again necessary to highlight that upper age limits have been imposed in virtually all of this work (even though many of these dysfunctions have been found to increase in prevalence with age). Therefore, the extent of both medically defined sexual dysfunction and personally defined sexual problems within older age groups remains unclear. The following discussion must be considered within this context.

Extent of sexual 'dysfunctions' among older people

As noted above, according to DSM-IV there are four, apparently discrete, types of sexual dysfunction that can be experienced: sexual desire disorders, sexual arousal disorders, orgasmic disorders, and sexual pain disorders. The following review aims to identify the prevalence of these disorders within the general population, and particularly among older people. Sexual dysfunctions within the context of chronic health problems are also briefly considered. These discussions will provide the background to an exploration of the impact of sexual problems upon individuals, and their relationships, central to which will be an elucidation of the role of age in this process.

While DSM-IV affords equal importance to each of the four sexual dysfunction categories mentioned above, this is certainly not the case within the published literature. Indeed, given the visibility of Viagra within the clinical and public imaginations, it is unsurprising that male erectile dysfunction is disproportionately represented within epidemiological surveys. As Marshall argues: 'The full and firm erection is generally viewed as the lynchpin on which the whole business of sex depends' (2002: 137). Inevitably therefore, women are under-represented in this body of work, although interest in 'female sexual dysfunction' has increased in recent years. The following review will briefly identify current evidence of rates of sexual dysfunction among men and women, focusing in particular upon key studies and those including older people.

Erectile dysfunction has been defined as the persistent inability to attain and/or maintain a penile erection sufficient to complete 'satisfactory' sexual intercourse (National Institute of Health 1992) (satisfactory for whom is unclear). Prevalence of erectile dysfunction will be explored initially through an examination of key surveys that have focused solely upon identifying the extent of this condition. The Massachusetts Male Aging Study (Feldman et al. 1994) is considered the most comprehensive survey of erectile dysfunction undertaken to date (Montosiri et al. 2002) and is notable for distinguishing between 'degrees' of dysfunction. In this study 1290 men aged 40–69 participated (53 per cent response rate) and the mean prevalence of erectile dysfunction was 52 per cent; 9.6 per cent of participants were classified as completely impotent, 25 per cent as moderately impotent, and 17.2 per cent as minimally impotent. Erectile dysfunction was most strongly associated with age – the prevalence of complete impotence ranged from 5.1 per cent among participants aged 40 to 15 per cent among participants aged 70. However, interestingly men in their sixties reported similar levels of satisfaction with their sex lives as men in their forties; this finding will be discussed in more detail in the following section. Adjusting for age effects revealed the following factors were associated with likelihood of erectile dysfunction: hypertension, heart disease, arthritis, diabetes, some medications and cigarette smoking.

Similar findings were reported by the 'Cologne Male Survey', however, this is worth considering separately because an older age group were included (Braun et al. 2000). Participants comprised 4489 men aged 30–80 who responded to a postal survey (56 per cent response rate) living in the Cologne area of Germany. A prevalence of erectile dysfunction of 19.2 per cent was reported, ranging from 2.3 per cent among men aged 30 to 39 to 15.7 per cent among men aged 50–59, 34.4 per cent among men aged 60–69 and 53.4 per cent among men aged 70–80. Again, interesting findings emerged in relation to age, with men aged 60 to 69 reporting the most dissatisfaction with their sex lives. There was an association between erectile dysfunction and hypertension, diabetes, pelvic surgery and urinary tract symptoms. There are many further studies exploring the prevalence of erectile dysfunction among older men; however, they report similar findings so they will not be included here. For comprehensive reviews of the prevalence of erectile dysfunction among older men see Kubin et al. (2003); Nicolosi et al. (2003); and Schiavi (1999).

The most widely cited generic sexual dysfunction survey was conducted in the USA (Laumann et al. 1999). This survey recruited 1749 women and 1410 men aged 18 to 59, and defined sexual dysfunction as experiencing one of the following seven 'problems' during the past 12 months: lacking desire for sex; arousal difficulties (i.e. erection problems in men, lubrication difficulties in women); inability achieving climax or orgasm; climaxing or ejaculating too rapidly; physical pain during intercourse; and not finding sex pleasurable. The last three 'problems' were only asked of people who were 'sexually active' in the last three months – the remainder were asked of people who reported a sexual partner during the past 12 months. Overall, 43 per cent of women and 31 per cent of men were found to be sexually 'dysfunctional'. The most common sexual problem experienced by women was lack of interest in sex (32 per cent for women aged 18–29; 27 per cent for women aged 50–59). All sexual problems decreased slightly for women with age, except for problems with lubrication. The most common sexual problem experienced by men was climaxing too early (30 per cent for men aged 18–29; 31 per cent for men aged 50–59). Increasing age for men was associated with experiencing erection difficulties and lacking desire for sex – men aged 50–59 were three times as likely to report erectile dysfunction and low sexual desire. There was an association between sexual dysfunction and impaired quality of life, although the direction of this association is unclear. The authors conclude that this 'first population-based assessment of sexual dysfunction in the half-century since Kinsey' indicates that sexual dysfunction warrants recognition as 'an important public health concern' (1999: 537).

Three UK population-based surveys of sexual dysfunction have been conducted. An anonymous postal survey of 798 men and 979 women aged 18 to 75 years (median age 50 years) identified erectile dysfunction (26 per cent) and premature ejaculation (14 per cent) as the most common sexual dysfunctions experienced by men; and vaginal dryness (28 per cent) and infrequent orgasm (27 per cent) as those most frequently reported by women (Dunn et al. 1998). Women were twice as likely as men to report that sexual intercourse was 'never or rarely a pleasant experience' (18 per cent women; 9 per cent men: 521). Erectile dysfunction and vaginal dryness were associated with increasing age (Dunn et al. 1999). For women, arousal, orgasmic and enjoyment 'problems' were predominantly associated with marital difficulties; however, no such association was identified for men.

Nazareth, Boynton and King (2003) report findings from a survey of 1065 women and 447 men aged 18–75 (mean age for women – 33, mean age for men – 36) recruited from 13 general practices in London. They identified a prevalence of sexual dysfunction of 22 per cent among men and 40 per cent among women. The most common dysfunctions reported were erectile dysfunction and 'lack or loss' of sexual desire in men and 'lack or loss' of sexual desire and 'failure of orgasmic response' in women. Interestingly, increasing age independently predicted sexual dysfunction among women, but not men.

Similar findings are reported from data gathered as part of the second *National Survey of Sexual Attitudes and Lifestyles* (Mercer et al. 2003), which included 11,161 men and women aged 16–44 years. Some 34.8 per cent of men and 53.8 per cent of women with at least one heterosexual partner during the last month reported a sexual problem during this period. Men most commonly reported lacking interest in sex (17 per cent), premature orgasm (12 per cent) and anxiety about performance (9 per cent); women most frequently reported inability to experience orgasm (14 per cent) and painful intercourse (12 per cent). Some 15.6 per cent of women and 6.2 per cent of men reported sexual problems which had lasted for at least six months in the past year. Unfortunately, given the low age cut-off of the sample, interesting data regarding the prevalence of these dysfunctions among people over 45 were not collected.

To conclude this section, the clear links between prevalence of sexual dysfunction and experience of chronic health conditions will be briefly explored. Although it is certainly not being proposed that these health conditions define the experience of most older people, they do increase in prevalence with age. While this is an area of the sexuality and ageing literature which is actually quite extensive, the majority draw on professional opinion rather than data gathered from older people themselves. Moreover, the impact of experiencing a sexual dysfunction on an older person (and potentially their partner) within the context of a chronic health condition remains largely unexamined.

Hill et al. (2003) report that, of 57 people with rheumatoid arthritis, over half felt that the pain and fatigue resulting from the condition limited their frequency of sexual intercourse. The ability to engage in intercourse was identified as important by 58 per cent of patients, but was found to decrease in importance with age. Similar findings emerged in a study of 63 couples where one partner was affected by heart failure (Westlake et al. 1999). Again, over half reported a decrease in sexual interest and 'sexual activity' (not defined) and for 30 per cent 'sexual relations' had ceased altogether. A review of the impact of diabetes on female sexuality identified that there is evidence that this condition can lead to decreased desire, pain on sexual intercourse and vaginal dryness (Enzil et al. 1998). As identified above, the prevalence of erectile dysfunction is also higher among men with diabetes (Feldman et al. 1994; Braun et al. 2000). Korpelainen et al. (1999) consider the literature on sexuality following a stroke, concluding that a stroke can result in decreased sexual interest, a marked increase in erectile dysfunction, diminished or absent vaginal lubrication and orgasmic difficulties. There is a large literature on the effect of cancer on sexuality – for example, Clark et al. (2003) report that a diagnosis of prostate cancer can lead to anxieties about physical intimacy and sexual performance, a loss of sexual interest, and changed relationships with partners. Similarly, breast cancer is known to lead to concerns about sexuality, for example, in relation to body image. However, while this is acknowledged as a problem for younger women, it often goes unrecognized for older women (Hordern 2000).

Sexuality within the context of cognitive impairment is regarded as a particularly 'knotty issue' (Sherman 1998: 141). Professional concerns are reflected in, and reinforced by, the fact much of the literature in this area highlights problems of 'inappropriate' or uncharacteristic sexual behaviours among people with dementia. However, the limited data available indicate that such behaviours are actually relatively rare. Burns et al. (1990), for example, found sexually inappropriate behaviour expressed among only 12 of 178 patients with dementia, with no differences by gender. Derouesne et al. (1996) report findings from a study which showed that, while 13 per cent of people with dementia of the Alzheimer's type experienced an increase in sexual activity, the remaining 87 per cent experienced a decrease in sexual activity. Therefore, while sexually 'disinhibited' behaviours can be expressed by a minority of people with dementia and may certainly represent a concern to their families and professional carers (see, for example, Archibald 2002), this aspect of sexuality within the context of dementia appears to be overplayed both within the literature, and in the context of professional beliefs. By contrast, little is known about the role that sex may play in maintaining intimacy when one partner is affected by cognitive impairment. Moreover, while we know an increasing amount about professional attitudes towards sexuality within the context of dementia, we know little about the views of the families of people with dementia or, indeed, the person with dementia themselves. However, addressing this knowledge gap is essential if we are to move from viewing the 'dementia victim' as an object of research, rather than a person in their own right (Cotrell and Shultz 1993).

Impact of sexual problems on older individuals

Little has been written about the specific impact of sexual dysfunctions on older people and, indeed, evidence of the extent to which such 'dysfunctions' constitute sexual problems at an individual level generally is sparse. This discussion is therefore largely theoretical and conclusions drawn in this section must be regarded as tentative.

One primary consideration in this discussion must be that sexuality has come to be seen as 'a property of the individual' (Giddens 1992: 175) and crucial to self-identity. That is not to say that sexual dysfunction must therefore automatically have a severe negative impact at an individual level, which is the message increasingly promoted within the popular media and the majority of the health and social care literature. Rather, the impact of experiencing such dysfunction is obviously highly complex, depending upon multiple factors including the nature and length of the dysfunction, gender, age and health status, past sexual experiences, the role and purpose of sex in an individual's life and normative expectations of sexual behaviour. However, the perceived centrality of sex to self-identity within contemporary society does mean that sexual 'failure' can have profound implications for the person affected. As Jackson and Scott (1997) remind us, being 'bad at sex' is not the same as being bad at gardening or golf.

Impact on older men

While it is recognized that erectile dysfunction is certainly not the only, or necessarily the most distressing, sexual problem men experience, it is the one about which most has been written and the only instance in which (albeit limited) information is available regarding the impact of sexual dysfunction upon older men (issues relating to how erectile dysfunction affects sexual partners will be discussed at the end of this section). Therefore, it will be taken as the focus of this discussion, although the need to explore experience of other sexual problems among older men must be recognized.

It has been argued that being 'bad at sex' is particularly difficult for men because 'in men, gender appears to "lean" on sexuality ... the need for sexual performance is so great' (Person 1980: 619). Indeed, the view of Zilbergeld (1992: 28) is very common, namely that: 'The man with an erection problem is a man in serious trouble ... His trouble stems not primarily from a penis that is not working up to expectation, but rather from the heavy symbolic baggage that he, and all of us, attach to the male organ.' Indeed, sexuality is considered central to current conceptions of masculinity (Tiefer 2000), resulting in erectile dysfunction being seen as a challenge to inherent masculinity (Person 1980) and a fate worse than death. The meaning of 'impotence', after all, goes way beyond specific genital malfunction to incorporate notions of powerlessness, weakness and 'feebleness of body' (*Oxford English Dictionary* 1989). Moreover, the centrality of (heterosexual) intercourse to modern understandings of sexuality places central responsibility for 'having sex' upon male sexual 'performance'.

It would therefore be expected that experiencing erectile dysfunction would have severe psychological consequences for the individual affected. There is limited evidence to suggest that such consequences can be profound. For example, the most common response among 40 men aged 22–72 years who had been prescribed Viagra for erectile dysfunction was a sense of emasculation (Tomlinson and Wright 2004) and the authors report that participants reactions were 'sometimes so severe that relationships, especially with their partners, were badly affected, often leading to depression' (2004: 1038).

However, the situation appears more complex when the experiences of older men are considered. In particular, there is an increasing body of evidence to suggest that age plays a crucial role in mediating the impact of erectile dysfunction upon an individual. Indeed, a number of studies report that, while erectile dysfunction increases in prevalence with age, the link between such dysfunction and variables such as depression and dissatisfaction with sex life becomes much less clear-cut among older men. The authors of the Massachusetts Male Aging Study, for example, report that:

> Despite the marked declines in actual events and behavior and in subjective aspects of sexuality, men in their sixties reported levels of satisfaction with their sex life and partners at about the same level as younger men in their forties.
>
> (McKinlay and Feldman 1994: 272)

Similarly, findings emerged from a survey of men aged 58–94 where older age was correlated with increased erectile dysfunction and decreased sexual activity, but a substantial number of older men reported continued active sexual behaviours and positive attitudes towards their own sexual ability (Bortz et al. 1999). In addition, Moore et al. (2003) looked specifically at age-effects within a sample of 560 men aged 19–87 attending a urology clinic for erectile difficulties, concluding that older men 'experience less difficulty' than younger men in adjusting to erectile dysfunction (2003: 381). Indeed, it was found that, while older men reported less positive ratings of their sex life and poorer erectile function than younger men, they also reported comparatively greater relationship satisfaction, less depressive symptomatology and more positive reactions from partners.

It is therefore apparent that (while obviously allowing for individual differences), overall older men appear to be less troubled by experiences of erectile dysfunction than younger men and continue to have satisfactory 'sex', supporting the idea that this may become less focused upon intercourse in later life (Gott and Hinchliff 2003a). Reasons for the differential impact of erectile dysfunction by age are suggested by qualitative data gathered from age diverse samples of men experiencing erectile dysfunction where normative expectations of sexual function by age emerge as crucial. Indeed, among a small sample of men aged over 50 experiencing erectile dysfunction, the challenge it represented to male self-identity varied by age (Gott and Hinchliff 2003b). For younger men erectile dysfunction was seen as abnormal and as such challenged masculinity, as Tiefer (2000) has argued. For example, one of the younger men in the sample experiencing erectile dysfunction viewed it as a threat to his inherent masculinity: 'I've lost confidence in it, of being able to perform like a normal man.' However, for men who defined themselves as 'old', erectile dysfunction was seen as expected and there was little evidence that it challenged their masculinity; indeed, it was considered 'normal' within the context of old age. As one participant in his seventies reported, he himself was not overly troubled by his experience of erectile dysfunction, but felt he would be if he were younger. Indeed, he was quite clear that 'There's something wrong with you if you're young and you can't [have an erection] ... (laughs) I should say you're ready for shooting if you're a young bloke and you can't manage it.'

The acceptance of erectile dysfunction as a 'natural' part of ageing is also suggested by data collected from interviews with 33 men and 27 women living in New Zealand. One male participant discusses his erectile dysfunction in a similar way to the above study participants:

> I think you've got to recognize that as you get older you've got less physical ability, you can't walk as far, as vigorously and the same with sex ... you've got to accept it, I don't treat it as negative because I think ... I just accept it as a fact.
>
> (Potts et al. 2004: 492)

The authors of the study argue that the view of erectile dysfunction as a 'pathology' which requires medical treatment is one outcome of the ways in which Viagra has been promoted and they note in particular that a number of their participants felt that the advent of this drug had led to older people feeling under increasing pressure to be sexually active.

The argument that erectile dysfunction is an expected and accepted feature of old age is also indicated by data indicating that this experience can represent a trigger to self-defining as an 'old person' (Daker-White and Donovan 2002), even among men in their fifties. This finding concurs with the theory that physical failings in later life can result in a 'Body Drop' (Mckee 1998), or transition in self-identity, through which an individual comes to think of himself or herself as someone who is old (McKee and Gott 2002). Therefore the psychological effects of erectile dysfunction among older men may relate more to their perceived loss of youth, than to the condition *per se*.

Within this context, emerging insights about the cultural dimensions of ageing indicate that this transition to 'old age' may be resisted and even postponed through the use of age-resisting technologies. The obvious example within this context is Viagra, which it is claimed, 'has rapidly bypassed its role as a treatment for specific pathologies to become the means for older men to 'reverse' their ageing and restore a synthetic youthful sexual performance that is widely seen as crucial to their self-esteem' (Gilleard and Higgs 2000: 77). However, data from the study mentioned above (Gott and Hinchliff 2003c) and presented in more detail in the final section of this chapter, indicate that, while some older men view Viagra as a means of staving off the transition to 'wearing slippers' (married man, aged 70), others see this new technology as interfering with the 'natural' progression of ageing. This indicates that a complex process is likely to mediate between the availability of 'age-resisting' technologies such as Viagra and their actual use.

It has been argued that the marketing of drugs such as Viagra has attempted to break down views of erectile dysfunction as a disease of old age in order to expand market potential (Tiefer 2000). One effect of this has been to promote the idea that while erectile dysfunction does increase with age, it is not caused by ageing, but rather is a specific pathology which can be medically treated at all ages (as discussed in more detail in Chapter 2). As such, Tiefer argues that a situation has been created where ageing provides no escape from the male sexual role. However, limited data available from older men themselves seem to indicate that, for this cohort of men in their sixties and upwards, erectile dysfunction is an expected part of ageing and accepted as such. That is not to say that it does not cause emotional distress, but rather that it seems to lead to less distress than it would for younger men where erectile function appears to be crucial to notions of masculinity. However, the creation and promotion of the myth of the 'sexy oldie', and notably within this context the availability of drugs to 'treat' sexual dysfunctions are likely to change this. It is probable therefore that for future cohorts of older men, the escape route of ageing will be blocked.

Impact of sexual problems on older women

If male sexuality is typically reduced to the mechanics of erectile function, women's sexuality is by contrast seen as emotional and complex. Female sexuality remains the 'dark continent' that Freud attempted, but failed, to demystify. Indeed, while the DSM-IV criteria for normal female sexuality breaks down the various components of 'female sexual dysfunction', we know very little about how these 'dysfunctions' are perceived and experienced by women themselves. Ultimately, we are left to reflect on the extent to which these actually represent problems to those women affected and, in particular, to older women affected in this way.

This section will briefly discuss the scant evidence available regarding the impact of sexual dysfunction upon women. The survey of sexual problems conducted by Dunn, Croft and Hackett and mentioned above, concluded that 'sexual problems cluster with self-reported physical problems in men, and with psychological and social problems in women' (1999: 144). In particular, they found that arousal problems, orgasmic dysfunction and inhibited enjoyment were strongly related to self-reported marital difficulties, as well as depression and anxiety. Dyspareunia (pain during intercourse) was associated with the presence of depression and marital difficulties. While they do not discuss these findings specifically, they are obviously not unexpected. However, what is unclear is which came first – the sexual dysfunction or the psychological problems and marriage difficulties. It seems safe to assume that all these factors are heavily inter-connected, but this remains empirically unexplored.

More revealing insights into how women experience sexual problems are provided by an interview study, which explored the impact of gynaecological and urological symptoms on 11 female participants aged 25–70 years old (Daker-White and Donovan 2002). In particular, there was evidence that sexual problems impact upon women's roles within a relationship and ultimately their feelings of femininity. For example, 'Kathy', a 40-year-old woman who was currently unable to have penetrative sex, talks about how this affected her relationship with her husband: 'he works hard and I think, "I can't even do that for him" and I feel a failure as a wife as well then, because I do love him' (2002: 101). Preliminary findings from a study interviewing women attending a psycho-sexual clinic in Sheffield support the view that, for many women, it is the impact upon their relationship, rather than the impact upon them individually, which is most significant in both defining, and seeking help for, a sexual problem (Gott and Hinchliff 2004). This issue is discussed in more detail in the next section.

Another interesting aspect of women's experiences of sexual problems which is evident in 'Kathy's' account is the fact that she makes little mention of her own pleasure. Similar findings have again been reported in our study (Gott and Hinchliff 2004). One woman, for example, talked about having sexual intercourse even when it caused her a lot of pain:

> Why do women have sex when it's painful? Maybe you want something for yourself … and I think you do want to please your partner, you don't want them to stray. It's like keeping the hook on the reel.
>
> (married participant, aged 43)

This reminds us that personal sexual satisfaction and pleasure are not the motivating factors for many women to have sex. This is likely to be particularly true for some older women for whom sex represented a marital duty, rather than a source of personal fulfilment (see Chapter 5). Any consideration of the circumstances under which sexual dysfunctions become sexual problems at an individual level must take this into account.

It is interesting to consider 'orgasmic dysfunction' within this context. A recent interview-based study conducted with 33 women aged 19–60 years identified that women are less concerned about having an orgasm during heterosexual intercourse than the sexological literature implies (Nicolson and Burr 2003). The authors conclude that:

> Women's notions of sexual desire and their constructions of their own sexuality informs the importance they ascribe to orgasm. Orgasm was something that was not expected. To expect orgasm would amount to a *pressure* on a man and a *demand* from a woman. Essentially, women considered their sexual desire as secondary to men's.
>
> (2003: 1743)

This finding again highlights the importance of contextualizing sex, both with regard to expectations of how men and women of different ages, sexual orientations, ethnicities, and so on, should behave sexually, as well as in relation to the role that sex can play between two people (as discussed in more detail below). Unfortunately, the effect of older age on women's experiences of sexual problems has not been elucidated to date and requires further attention.

Indeed, to conclude, it seems fundamental that research is conducted which goes beyond identifying the prevalence of certain medically definable sexual dysfunctions to explore the extent to which these represent real problems at an individual level. Given claims that many of these dysfunctions increase in prevalence of age, there is obviously a need, not only to include older people in studies of this type, but also to consider how both age and cohort affect the perception and experience of sexual dysfunctions.

Impact of sexual problems upon sexual relationships

As previously discussed, a key criticism of the DSM-IV classification of sexual problems has been its neglect of the relational context of sexuality (The Working Group for a New View of Women's Sexual Problems 2001). Indeed, while we know little about the impact of sexual problems on older people individually, we know even less about the impact of such problems upon their relationships. However, this must be considered crucial given that, first, most older people are sexually active primarily within the context of a long-term relationship and, second, previous research has highlighted the importance of attending to the relationship impact of sexual problems. Indeed, it is increasingly apparent that defining sexual dysfunctions solely in relation to specific genital function with the aim of orgasm is far too simplistic. Sex does not merely consist of intercourse, and does not only occur as a means of deriving pleasure.

Daker-White and Donovan (2002: 106) argue that 'sexual activity is perhaps best understood as a form of "transaction" of intimacy between partners within a relationship fundamentally understood as being mutual in aim and intent'. Their study exploring the impact of sexual dysfunction concluded that: 'Peoples' lives can apparently be turned upside down when they are unable to engage in what is evidently the primary defining feature of an intimate heterosexual relationship: penetrative sexual intercourse' (2002: 106). Preliminary findings from our study with women experiencing sexual problems confirm the centrality of sexual intercourse to many (heterosexual) intimate relationships (Gott and Hinchliff 2004). As discussed above, a common trigger to seeking treatment was the belief that not doing could lead to relationship disintegration because male partners would not be involved in a non-sexual relationship. This participant's comments were fairly typical:

> At night I would have him saying, "Oh, it's natural, everybody does it, come on and get on with it, it's here to be enjoyed, there's something wrong with you if you don't enjoy it" and I just absolutely hated it ... I just thought I can't go on like this, something's got to give, either our marriage was going to split up or I've got to change.
>
> (married participant, aged 38)

However, there is again evidence that age mediates the impact of sexual problems at a relationship level. For example, findings from research with people aged > 70 years who had been married for at last 22 years indicates that, for people of this age involved in a long-term relationship, sex may assume less importance (Hinchliff and Gott 2004). Indeed, even though participants reported that penetrative sex had played an important role in all their marriages, no significant negative effects were reported in terms of relationship stability when this was no longer possible. When asked about this, responses such as 'Oh no. It's something that you haven't got to have' (male participant, aged 79) and 'We are quite happy as we are. We get round it' (female participant, aged 72) were elicited. Adapting to this change in their relationship involved maintaining intimacy in other ways, for example, through touching and hugging. For instance, one participant commented that her husband's erectile dysfunction did not bother her overly because: 'As you get older I don't think a sexual relationship as such is as important as a love and cuddle', (female participant, aged 72).

Attending to the impact of a sexual problem on a relationship rather than just concentrating upon the effect on an individual therefore appears crucial for people of all ages. As such, drugs used to treat sexual dysfunctions obviously need to be considered within the same context, although little research has examined this issue to date. One of the only studies to do so was undertaken in New Zealand and focused on the 'downside of Viagra' (Potts et al. 2003: 697) in interviews with 27 female partners of men who had been prescribed the drug to treat their erectile dysfunction. Participants expressed concerns that they had not been involved in consultations when Viagra was prescribed and had not received information about the drug. In addition, some participants reported 'unwelcome' (2003: 703) changes to their sexual relationships and, in particular, talked about a shift in focus away from foreplay to intercourse, as well as the pressure they felt under to have intercourse so as to 'make the most of the tablet' (2003: 705). Interesting findings emerged in relation to age. In particular, some of the older women in the sample reported that they felt it was 'natural' to have less sex in later life and their partner's use of Viagra not only reversed this natural process, but also led to them having doubts about their own sexual desires. For example, one 60-year-old woman stated that: 'I think Viagra has made a lot of people feel inadequate ... everybody's on the defensive about how often they have sex and so on, in the older age group' (cited Potts et al. 2003: 712). This finding indicates that the 'sexy oldie' stereotype discussed in Chapter 2 has resulted in a shift in older people's beliefs about sex within the context of ageing and, in particular, resulted in pressure to be sexually active in later life.

Older people's experiences of seeking treatment for sexual problems

The final section of this chapter will explore older people's experiences of seeking treatment for a sexual problem. The limited evidence available regarding treatment-seeking within this context will be reviewed initially and data will then be presented looking at the attitudes of a small sample of older people experiencing sexually-related concerns.

There is evidence that the majority of people of all ages who experience a sexual problem never seek treatment for this. A survey of the prevalence of sexual problems among 1768 adults, for example, found that 49 per cent (n = 281) of male respondents and 39 per cent (n = 293) of female respondents would like to seek help for sexual problems, but only 4–6 per cent of these participants had actually done so (Dunn et al. 1998). Patient barriers to discussing sexual problems within medical consultations remain relatively unexplored, although a study undertaken with women aged 40–80 with Type II diabetes (Sarkadi and Rosenqvist 2001) identified that participants felt uncomfortable raising these problems with a medical doctor and only one participant reported having had sexual issues raised with her by her doctor. The following barriers to initiating discussions about sexual issues were identified: age and gender of the GP, sexual issues being a specialist rather than a generalist area, and a lack of time and privacy in consultations.

It also appears that older people may be even more reluctant to seek treatment for a sexual problem than younger people. For example, as noted in the previous chapter, older people who suspect they have a sexually transmitted infection have been found to delay longer between symptom recognition and clinical presentation than younger people (Gott et al. 1999). Barriers reported to seeking treatment among this group of symptomatic patients aged > 50 years included wanting to 'wait and see' if symptoms improved and being embarrassed or afraid to seek treatment. However, overall, little is known about older people's help-seeking behaviours for sexually-related concerns.

The following section reports findings from a qualitative, interview-based study conducted with 45 people aged 50 to 92 recruited at random from one general practice surgery in Sheffield (as discussed in Chapter 3). In-depth, semi-structured interviews explored key issues relating to sexuality and ageing, including attitudes towards, and experience of seeking treatment for sexual problems. Moreover, although it was not our aim in this study to recruit older people with a sexual problem, 25 participants reported current, or recent, experience of such a problem. Ten participants reported personal experience of erectile dysfunction (seven men and three women whose partners were experiencing, or had experienced, erectile dysfunction). Seven older women had experienced reduced vaginal lubrication and one man talked about his female partner's experience of this. Reduced lubrication was reported as a 'symptom' of the menopause and as making it difficult, or impossible, to have intercourse. Four participants (two women and two men) reported direct experience of reduced libido attributed to hysterectomy and four participants reported specific medical diagnoses as interfering directly with their personal sexual health, including cardiac problems and arthritis. Only six of these participants had sought help for their problems – two participants with erectile dysfunction, two regarding hysterectomy and one regarding vaginal dryness. No participant reported that their GP had initiated a discussion about sexual issues with them, even when conditions were diagnosed (and related medications prescribed) with a known impact on sexual health.

Preferred source of treatment

Participants were asked where they would seek treatment if they experienced a sexual problem. All cited the GP as their preferred source of help if in this situation, relating this to a number of factors, including having a good relationship with their GP and satisfaction with past consultations:

Int: If you did need to go for ... any help with sexual problems, would you know where to go?

P: Well, I think I should come straight to my family doctor, me, I mean, I've confidence in him, to come and have a talk to him, he would advise me, in fact I've no doubt he would. I've a lot of confidence in [name of doctor].

(married male participant, aged 77)

This finding confirms that the GP is seen as an appropriate source of help if a sexual problem is experienced (Read et al. 1997; Dunn et al. 1998). However, primary care was also preferred because most participants were not aware of any other sources of help and, as explored below, those participants with experience of sexual problems found these difficult to discuss with their GP and most had not done so.

Barriers to seeking treatment

Despite the GP being seen to be the most appropriate source of help if sexual problems were experienced, significant barriers were considered to exist to seeking treatment in primary care settings. These included the demographic characteristics of the GP, GP attitudes towards later life sexuality, the attribution of sexual problems to 'normal ageing', shame/embarrassment and fear, perceiving sexual problems as 'not serious' and lack of knowledge about appropriate services.

GP characteristics

Several participants expressed preferences to consult a GP of a specific gender or age about sexual health issues. Overall, there was a preference for consultations with a GP with similar demographic characteristics to the participants:

P: I would see the male doctor rather than the lady doctor, I find it easier to talk to him about things ... The doctors must get a lot of that sort of thing and the older the doctor the better, young doctors probably have difficulties I think, but if the doctor's a bit older, he has been through the mill himself and he could probably help better.

Int: Do you think he would have more understanding of what's going on?

P: I think so, yes. Well, they would have personal knowledge, really; of course they are human as well, aren't they doctors? I mean [name of doctor] told me he has got five kids, it's nothing to be ashamed of.

(widowed male participant, aged 80)

Preferences to consult a GP of a similar age and gender were underpinned by the desire to minimize embarrassment through discussing sexual concerns with someone they felt was likely to have had similar experiences as themselves. This finding is consistent with previous studies which have identified that most people prefer consultations about sexual issues with a health professional of the same gender and age as themselves (Stokes and Mears 2000; Sarkadi and Rosenqvist 2001) and that the personal characteristics of the GP can represent a barrier to treatment seeking.

Age related factors
The perceived attitude of the GP towards an older person seeking help for a sexual problem was cited as a barrier to treatment seeking, notably by two men currently experiencing erectile dysfunction. Such concerns were expressed within the context of having built up a relationship with their GP over a number of years.

> Int: Yes, you have seen him [GP about erectile dysfunction]?
> P: No, I've contemplated seeing him, but I just don't know how much importance the doctor would attach to it, you know what I mean? I mean, getting to our age, he says it's about time you packed up anyway [laughs]. You know what I mean, I don't want him to think I'm a sex maniac or anything like that.
>
> (married male participant, aged 65)

> I just don't know what [name of doctor] would think about it if I came down to see him [about my erectile dysfunction].
>
> (married male participant, aged 81)

The stereotype of the 'asexual older people' was also seen as inhibiting treatment seeking in other ways. In particular, for this generation of older people, sex was discussed as something that was often considered private: 'A lot of older people I think don't go to the doctors if they experience problems because they think it is something that should be kept quiet ... [they] live with it instead of seeking some sort of help' (divorced female participant, aged 62).

Moreover, age also presented a barrier to treatment-seeking as sexual problems attributed to ageing were seen as 'normal' and irreversible. This led participants to feel that suitable treatments would not be available, or appropriate.

> I think the older you get the more difficult it is to seek advice because when you're younger things should be right and if they are not then it's almost automatic to look for the remedy. I think as you get older if things aren't right then maybe it's because you're getting old.
>
> (married female participant, aged 73)

While comparable data regarding treatment-seeking for sexual problems among older people are not available, there is evidence that attributing symptoms to normal ageing can inhibit treatment for conditions such as urinary tract infections in later life (Cunningham-Burley et al. 1996).

A further set of barriers to presenting with sexual problems related to age were reported by older men experiencing erectile dysfunction. First, there was a common belief that younger men were more entitled to drugs such as Viagra than men of their age, particularly given awareness of the limited resources of the NHS to fund these medications: 'If there were plenty around [Viagra] to serve these people that's youngcr, that's the time of your life, you know, I would like to take it, but I wouldn't want to join the queue before younger people' (married male participant, aged 81).

In addition, concerns were expressed about the side-effects of Viagra, particularly given that many participants had been diagnosed with cardiac problems. Finally, for one male participant, Viagra was seen as 'artificial', interfering with the 'natural' progression of old age: 'We accept the fact that we are what we are and it's interfering with nature' (married man, aged 74).

'Severity' of sexual problems

The perception that sexual problems were not a 'severe' health problem also deterred treatment-seeking: 'It's something to do with life's pleasure that, it's something that's not really serious, it is in a way, but it's not damaging your health' (married male participant, aged 81). This consideration was made within the context of concerns about GP workload and also related to participants' experiences of having to pay for medical care prior to the advent of the NHS.

Psychosocial factors

Psychosocial factors were cited by participants as presenting a barrier to treatment-seeking within the context of sexual problems, including shame, embarrassment and fear. The experience of shame was related to societal attitudes towards sex, particularly among older people: 'I think sex is a thing that is very much pushed under the carpet and we don't talk about it, we are ashamed to talk about it, it isn't something you go to your doctors for' (single, divorced female participant, aged 66). Similarly, sex was also seen to be an embarrassing topic: 'Just the fact you can't maintain an erection, I find that a little bit embarrassing … you're just a little bit inhibited as to what you come and see your doctor about, aren't you?' (married male participant, aged 65).

Fear of the potential underlying cause of a sexual problem was also noted as having an impact upon decisions to seek treatment. This was particularly notable within the context of erectile dysfunction where some participants had awareness of the association between this condition and prostate cancer: 'I tend to be fearful in case there might be something wrong … I heard it on the radio, 10,000 men and I worked it out, that's 200 a week die from prostate cancer and you think, is it me in that clump?' (married male participant, aged 70).

Lack of knowledge about services/lack of appropriate services

Service-related issues were mentioned by several female participants, notably within the context of a desire to seek treatment in an anonymous setting to minimize potential embarrassment and shame as discussed above. One older woman felt strongly that genitourinary medicine clinics, which she refers to as 'sex clinics', should be widely available to people of all ages:

I think sex clinics are a damn good idea, I think they should perhaps make people a little more aware of them … I think people do know of them but not much about them, I think there needs to be a lot more general knowledge about it and I think it should be made very apparent that it's for people of all ages.

(married female participant, aged 73)

However, other participants associated genitourinary medicine clinics with 'VD clinics' and felt there was still a lot of stigma attached to seeking treatment within this setting.

Conclusion

This small qualitative study identified that, although older people see the GP as the most appropriate professional to discuss sexual problems with, they rarely initiate such discussions themselves. These findings confirm and extend previous research, which has identified that a significant proportion of people who experience sexual problems do not seek treatment for these (Dunn et al. 1998). They also confirm that sexual problems are perceived as embarrassing and potentially shameful and inhibit treatment-seeking for this reason. This has also been reported in relation to treatment-seeking for STIs among both younger (Leenaars et al. 1993) and older people (Gott et al. 1999).

However, that older age can represent a barrier to seeking treatment for sexual problems in other ways has not previously been reported. The recognition among older participants that sex in later life does not meet with societal expectations and therefore may be disapproved of by their GP is interesting, particularly given evidence which will be presented in the next chapter that GPs draw upon similar stereotypes of later life sexuality when making judgements as to whether it is appropriate to raise sexual issues with older patients (Gott et al. 2004).

This chapter has explored the prevalence and experience of sexual problems among older people. Initially, accepted definitions of sexual dysfunction were considered and found to be highly problematic. In addition, it was noted that, although the prevalence of certain sexual dysfunctions has been claimed to increase with age, the impact these have on older people themselves remains largely unexplored. However, evidence was identified that age plays a crucial factor in determining the experience of a sexual problem, although this requires further investigation. Finally, difficulties that older people experience in seeking treatments for sexual problems were examined. Having identified the significant barriers that older people experience in discussing sexual problems with a health professional, a key recommendation to arise from this work was that professionals need to adopt a more proactive role in this area. Reasons why this role is not adopted, and the barriers that health professionals themselves experience in discussing sexual issues with older people, are the focus of the next chapter.

Acknowledgements

Extracts from this chapter are based on the following article and are reproduced with the permission of Oxford University Press: Gott, M. and Hinchliff, S. (2003) Barriers to seeking treatment for sexual problems in primary care: a qualitative study with older people, *Family Practice*, 20(6): 690–5.

8

Health professionals' views on later life sexuality and sexual health

> Doctors are not much good at talking about sex because doctors are people and people are not much good at talking about sex. In no other area of medicine does our own guilt, fear and personal experience so affect the consultation and our ability to help.
>
> (Tate 2000: 100)

Introduction

While the increasing 'sexualization' (Hawkes 1996) of contemporary society may make us feel as though we are 'surrounded' by sex, for most people, sex remains an intensely private affair. Indeed, although sex may be talked about more than ever before and it is now possible to read details of 'celebrity' sex lives in the Sunday papers, discussions about personal sexual behaviours tend to take place only between close friends. In everyday life, few people ask us directly about our own sexual experiences and magazine problem pages attest to the fact that sex can be difficult to discuss, even with sexual partners. It is therefore unsurprising that people, whether adopting the role of 'professional' or 'patient', consider sex to be a difficult topic to discuss in health care consultations.

Indeed, despite the increasing role defined for health professionals in sexual health management and, in particular, in later life sexual health management, sexual issues are known to be particularly problematic to address within a clinical context. While the (arguably inappropriate) rhetoric may be that health professionals should be advising older people about how to have more and better sex as a means to improve their overall well-being, the reality seems very different. This chapter will explore the evidence available regarding health professional management of later life sexual health concerns, drawing in particular upon findings from a qualitative study undertaken with GPs and practice nurses working in Sheffield. Prior to examining the attitudes and experiences of these study participants, the discussion will consider the difficulties posed by discussing a 'private' topic such as sexuality within a patient consultation. Evidence regarding the barriers that are experienced in discussing sexual issues with patients of all ages will be drawn from research conducted with both doctors and nurses. The study findings will enable the additional barriers that inhibit discussions with older patients to be explored. In concluding this section it will be argued that, while there is evidence that health professionals should be involved in discussions with older people about sexual health issues, more realistic recommendations about professional involvement in this area are needed. These need to be tailored to real-life clinical situations and recognize training requirements and constraints of time within the typical consultation. Finally, it will be argued that the limits of medical and nursing responsibility with regard to later life sexual health management need careful consideration.

Discussing sex with patients of all ages within the consultation

While the link between good sex and good health provides the backdrop for an increasing raft of recommendations about how health professionals should manage patient's sexual health concerns, the reality appears to be very different. Humphrey and Nazareth (2001), for example, found that among 133 London GPs, only 8 had a special interest in sexual health and only 46 had received postgraduate training in taking a sexual history. Most GPs identified more than one barrier to discussing sexual concerns in consultations and key barriers included lack of training/education/knowledge, fear of opening a 'floodgate' and their own embarrassment. The level of education these study participants report does not seem atypical given that training for doctors in managing sexual health at both undergraduate and postgraduate levels has been deemed inadequate (Adler 1998; Skelton and Matthews 2001). Lack of training has also been identified as inhibiting discussions of sexual risk behaviours among Dutch GPs (Verhoeven et al. 2003), where it was identified as a barrier to undertaking sexual counselling by nearly 70 per cent of the 122 study participants.

Further barriers identified in this study included language and comprehension problems (74 per cent), ethnic differences (68 per cent) and age difference between doctor and patient (31 per cent). The doctor–patient relationship appeared to have an interesting impact upon the likelihood of mentioning sexual issues, with a close professional relationship with a patient cited as a barrier to initiating such discussions by 71 per cent of GPs, and a patient visiting for the first time as a barrier by 60 per cent of participants. Doctor–specific barriers identified in this study included finding it difficult to raise sexual issues with patients who have no genital complaints (79 per cent), time constraints (61 per cent) and not feeling familiar enough with certain sexual practices (for example, among gay patients). Overall, about one-fifth of participants stated that they regularly felt uncomfortable when taking a sexual history, and 31 per cent were concerned that sexually-related questions might be regarded as intrusive by their patients.

It has been argued that nurses may be better placed than doctors to manage patients' sexual health concerns. For example, Baraniak et al. (2002: 166) propose that: 'Patients feel they can relate better to a nurse as an equal. For this reason they may be able to communicate their needs more readily.' This ease of communication is likely to be especially important for 'difficult' topics such as those related to sexuality. The 'holistic' philosophy shaping nursing practice has also been argued to result in sexual health being afforded higher priority by nursing staff and as being conceptualized in broad psychosocial, rather than purely medical, terms (Guthrie 1999). Hoolaghan and Blache (1993) have also suggested a number of additional reasons why nurses may be better equipped than doctors to discuss sexual health issues with patients including: nurses having more responsibility for health promotion; nurses often having longer consultations; and tasks carried out by nurses often being more involved than those carried out by doctors and therefore including more time for communication.

However, it is acknowledged that nurses can also experience considerable barriers to discussing sexual health issues with patients and do not address sexuality routinely (Wilson and Williams 1988). Indeed, Waterhouse and Metcalfe (1991) argue that nurses will only discuss sexual issues if the patient initiates such a discussion. This is supported by empirical data gathered from oncology nurses (Wilson and Williams 1988) and staff nurses working in acute surgical wards (Guthrie 1999). These findings fit with the traditional perceived role of the nurse and the fact that, historically, the nurses' own sexuality has been 'suppressed and repressed with the aim of purity and asexuality' (Griffith 1990: 34). This has been reflected in nursing teaching, where sexual health has only recently been introduced into the curriculum and has been described as being taught with a narrow focus (Weston 1993). Heath and White (2002) collate the literature regarding sexuality and nursing to identify numerous factors as influencing the integration of sexuality within nursing practice (Table 8.1).

Research conducted specifically with practice nurses has identified further barriers to addressing sexual health issues in UK primary care settings (Stokes and Mears 2000). Two hundred and thirty four practice nurses who participated in a questionnaire survey identified the following key barriers: lack of time (64 per cent), lack of training (61 per cent) and concerns about not being able to cope with the issues raised by the patient (53 per cent). This study also found that practice nurses felt more comfortable discussing sexual health issues with female patients and teenagers, than with male patients and those of different sexual orientations (Stokes and Mears 2000). This finding has been reported elsewhere where it was attributed to nurses developing stereotyped images of certain patient groups (Guthrie 1999).

Table 8.1 Factors that appear to adversely affect the integration of sexuality within nursing practice

Individual practitioner factors
Biographical factors e.g. formal practice of religion (Payne 1976; Lewis and Bor 1994; White 1994); family upbringing: traditional (negative) attitudes to sex (Hacker 1984; White 1994; Guthrie 1999)
Restrictive views on sexuality: e.g. contraception, masturbation (Hacker 1984; Webb 1988)
Ageist stereotypes of 'asexual' older people (Webb 1988; White 1994)
Heterosexist assumptions or restrictive views on homosexuality (Hacker 1984; White 1994; Guthrie 1999)
Embarrassment in discussion of sexual issues (Lawler 1991; Wall-Haas 1991; White 1994; Guthrie 1999; Meerabeau 1999)
Discomfort in consideration of sex within the context of altered states of health: e.g. disability, mental illness, life-limiting illness (Hacker 1984; White 1994)
Not perceived by nurse as a priority for patient/focus of treatment (Kautz et al. 1990; White 1994; Guthrie 1999)
Nurse perception of patient discomfort in considering sexuality issues (Hacker 1984; Kautz et al. 1990; White 1994)
Lack of theoretical knowledge about sexual issues (Payne 1976; Webb 1988; Wall-Haas 1991; Matocho and Waterhouse 1993; Lewis and Bor 1994; White 1994)
Organizational/practice setting factors
Lack of privacy (Lewis and Bor 1994; White 1994; Guthrie 1999)
Lack of time (Lewis and Bor 1994; White 1994; Guthrie 1999)

Source: Cited in Heath and White (2002: 245)

Sex, health care and older people

Very little is known about health care professional attitudes towards discussing sexual issues with older patients. While anecdotal evidence indicates that older age is likely to introduce a further set of barriers to discussing an already complex issue within the context of a patient consultation, this represents an under-researched area. Indeed, it was the aim of the study presented below to address this gap in current knowledge by eliciting the views and experiences of GPs and practice nurses regarding later life sexual health management. Prior to examining key findings from this study, factors theorized to influence professional attitudes towards discussing sexual issues with older people will be briefly discussed.

As Lupton recognizes (1994: 123): 'While medicine is predicated on scientific principles of objectivity and the ethical tenet of altruism, moral values are suffused throughout the medical encounter.' Moreover, there are few areas in which medicine's role as moral arbiter has been more sharply defined than in relation to sexuality. Foucault (1979) states that medicine has replaced religion as the guiding force in the definition and regulation of 'normal' and 'abnormal' sexualities, and in the last chapter the continuing influence of medicine upon sexuality was evident in discussions of 'sexual dysfunctions'. The extent to which individual practitioners adopt the role of 'moral arbiter' is unknown, although their own attitudes towards sexuality are certainly recognized to influence their sexual health management. Indeed, the need for health professionals to first of all recognize, and subsequently 'put aside' personal attitudes towards the morality of various sexual activities is stressed within the sexual health training literature (Curtis et al. 1995).

Within this context, the extent to which health professionals subscribe to, and are subsequently influenced by, societal representations of sexuality and ageing is certainly pertinent. While little evidence is available from health professionals themselves, research discussed in the previous chapter identified that older people do feel that professionals may perceive them as asexual. The example of a married man in his sixties was cited, where concerns that his GP would think he should have 'packed up' sex and was a 'sex maniac', inhibited him from discussing his erectile difficulties. The study also identified that health professionals were not discussing sex with this older age group, even when diagnosing conditions or prescribing medications with a known effect on sexual health. Similar findings have been reported by a Swedish study exploring sexual health management among 33 women aged 40–80 with Type II diabetes where only one participant had had sexual health issues raised with her by her doctor (Sarkadi and Rosenqvist 2001). Although little is known about how older people would react to being asked about sexual health concerns, a North American study indicates that most are likely to see this as appropriate, and potentially welcome, within the right context (Loehr et al. 1997).

Indeed, the accounts of older people presented in the previous chapter indicate that by not mentioning sexual issues, health professionals can reinforce the view that sex is not an appropriate concern in later life. However, many professionals may perceive older people as being 'of a generation' who do not perceive sexual issues as legitimate areas of discussion within a medical encounter. For example, Cranston and Thin (1998) write that professionals may have difficulties discussing sexual issues with older patients because they are likely to have grown up with the idea that sex is 'improper'. Nevertheless, the extent to which this view is underpinned by professional experiences of having discussed sex with older people remains unclear.

The lack of evidence regarding current practice in later life sexual health management has not prevented the publication of a raft of recommendations advocating the greater involvement of health professionals in the proactive discussion of sexual issues with older people. Heath and White (2002: 144), for example, recommend that health care professionals create an 'environment which "gives permission" for [older] individuals to feel comfortable in raising [sexual] issues of concern'. Kessel goes further, arguing that 'Professionals should advise that sex is good for ... [older people] and orgasm achieved by masturbation may relieve anxiety and promote well-being'

(2001: 122). She views professional responsibility as not only to manage specific sexual health concerns, but also to provide advice on 'spicing up the sex life' (2001: 123). The issue of where health professional responsibility for later life sexual health management ends will be considered in the conclusion to this chapter.

The context of the study – why focus on primary care?

Within a UK context, the health professionals with the most opportunity to initiate discussions of sexual health issues with older people are those working within primary care. GPs and practice nurses represent the first point of contact for many people with sexual health concerns and would be expected to be a particularly appropriate source of help for middle-aged and older people who are frequent attenders to primary care (National Statistics 1998). Moreover, this setting has been identified as an appropriate place to seek treatment for sexual health concerns by patients of all ages. Read, King and Watson (1997), for example, found that 70 per cent of a sample of 170 patients attending a general practice thought that the GP was an appropriate source of help if sexual health concerns were experienced. Similar findings were reported following an anonymous postal questionnaire survey (n = 1768), where the GP was the preferred source of professional help for sexual problems (Dunn et al. 1998). The GP has also been identified as the preferred source of help for older people if sexual health concerns are experienced (Gott and Hinchliff 2003c).

The role of primary care in sexual health management has been given prominence by the *National Sexual Health Strategy* (Department of Health 2001a), which identified an 'expanded role' for GPs and practice nurses in this area. However, the Royal College of General Practitioners report that sexual health issues 'are often not addressed' (1995: xiii) in primary care consultations. The role of the practice nurse in primary care has achieved increasing importance in recent years, with the number of nurses based in GP surgeries reaching 24,959 in Britain by 2003 (DoH 2003; Information Services NHS Scotland 2003). In relation to sexual health specifically, the importance of nurses has been highlighted. *The National Sexual Health Strategy*, for example, states that: 'The role of nurses in this field is expanding' (DoH 2001a: 24), as reflected in an intention to appoint nurse specialists and nurse consultants in sexual health (2001a).

With regards to older people, the review above highlighted that little research has been conducted exploring health professional attitudes towards later life sexual health management, particularly within the context of primary care. We conducted a study with GPs and practice nurses recruited from diverse primary care practices within Sheffield, UK to address this gap in current knowledge and our key findings are presented below.

Methods

The study methodology is described in more detail elsewhere (Gott et al. 2004; Gott and Hinchliff 2004). To summarize, in-depth, semi-structured interviews were conducted with 35 practice nurses and 22 GPs recruited from socio-economically diverse general practice surgeries in Sheffield in the North of England. Potential participants were identified from all primary care practices within Sheffield and purposive sampling was used to maximize diversity of participant and practice characteristics. This involved stratified sampling according to practice type, including single-handed practices, single sex practices and mixed sex practices and across the four Sheffield Primary Care Trusts. GP participants were also stratified by gender. Interviews with GPs were conducted between November 2002 and April 2003 and with practice nurses between August and October 2003. The interviews were transcribed verbatim and the data analysed thematically. First, transcripts were read individually in order to become familiar with the content and preliminary notes were made on potential themes. Each transcript was then loaded into NUD*IST and further analysed to develop more thematic categories, which encompassed all the issues raised by participants and explored in the interviews.

Findings

Previous reports from this research have discussed barriers participants experienced in discussing sexual issues with patients of all ages (Gott et al. 2004), and that GP participants experienced in discussing sex with patients of the opposite sex (Hinchliff et al. 2004b) and with non-heterosexual patients (Hinchliff et al. 2004a). The study findings reported here consider the extent to which older age impeded discussions of sexual issues within GP and practice nurse consultations and will be discussed in relation to the following key areas: participants' definitions of sexual health; professional role in later life sexual health management; raising sexual issues with older patients; and barriers to discussing sexual health with older patients.

What is 'sexual health'?

When speaking about day-to-day clinical practice, participants acknowledged a tendency to equate sexual health with younger age groups and a relatively small number of issues relating to preventing pregnancy (and particularly teenage pregnancy) and STIs:

> the sort of thing [sexual health] conjures up in my mind is more to do with younger people really, and safe sex and sensible practice. It's often something we don't really think about for middle-aged people, probably something that's very much overlooked, I would think.
>
> (practice nurse, aged 40–49)

This attitude was reflected in the impact that age was seen to have upon discussions of sexual health issues within consultations: 'Discussion of sexuality will be peaking in late teens, early twenties, there are some understandable reasons for that, but logically we should be having it as a thread throughout others' lives' (female GP, aged 40–49). The link participants made between sexual health, sexual risk-taking and younger people is not unsurprising given that it reflects UK sexual health policy. Indeed, as discussed in Chapter 6, the most recent policy document published by the Department of Health (2001a) explicitly aims to reduce the rates of STIs among *younger* people. While most participants felt that such policy documents did not have a significant influence upon their day-to-day working, it is apparent that STIs and younger people are not only prioritized at a policy level, but also by individual practitioners.

Focusing more specifically upon the role of sexual health within medical and nursing care, an interesting distinction arose. Nurse participants regarded sexual health to form part of holistic nursing care and, as such, as an important aspect of their role: 'If we're going to look after people as a whole then that [sex] is part of it, part of life and we can't ignore it' (practice nurse, aged 30–39). This sentiment reflects discussions regarding the role of nurses within sexual health management and the 'whole person' philosophy that underpins much nursing training (Guthrie 1999). By contrast, some GPs expressed concerns about whether sexual health was actually a 'medical' issue or not:

> Again, thinking about issues that you have raised, how much of this is health-related, how much of it is outside our sphere all together and should we be trying to influence things which are especially outside our control and more particularly outside our gift? I think it's one of the things that was very clearly highlighted when Viagra did become available, it was something very accessible and, all of a sudden, it seemed to be creating a demand which was previously not seen as a health problem at all, it was seen as a social problem or a relationship problem or whatever, but not specifically to do with doctors and nurses and all of a sudden it was, it was, like, taking over that area. Are we the appropriate people to be doing it? Should we be doing it?
>
> (male GP, aged 40–49)

This account indicates that the unease about the medicalization of sexuality, which has surfaced in debates on 'female sexual dysfunction' and NHS provision of drugs such as Viagra, is also experienced by individual medical practitioners.

Professional role in later life sexual health management

Participants were aware that they could assume a 'permission granting' role for older people in relation to sexuality, first by being proactive in mentioning sexual issues. As a practice nurse participant identified:

> It's even more difficult to talk about sex, the older you are, because people see sex as something that young nubile bodies do, not aged, wrinkly, fat or thin bodies do and it's almost as if it's a real no-no. You can't admit that you are sexually active because you're not young and beautiful. You couldn't be on one of these programmes that they have on the tele, showing your bosom to everybody, you know, [whispers] you can't be having sex, and the fact that some of the most satisfying sex

a lot of people have is when they are older, more confident, less frightened of things, is completely ignored by almost everybody and I think actually putting that into words to some people empowers them to realize that they can ask for that, it isn't something that they should be denied.

(practice nurse, aged 60–69)

This supports Heath and White (2002: 144), who recommend that health care professionals create an 'environment which "gives permission" for [older] individuals to feel comfortable in raising [sexual] issues of concern'. However, as will become evident in the subsequent discussion, this role was infrequently adopted by participants in this study.

A more complex aspect of the 'permission granting' role was apparent in GPs' accounts. Indeed, when they were asked to reflect upon their role in later life sexual health management, it became clear that this extended beyond the strictly 'medical' to incorporate wider issues of helping patients to define 'normal' and 'appropriate' sexualities. In this situation, they felt older people perceived them to be moral arbiters who could not only provide information about the effects of physiological ageing upon sexuality, but could also judge the appropriateness of remaining sexually active into later life, particularly within the context of forming a new sexual relationship following divorce or widowhood. As one GP participant identified:

I think they are informed of the stereotype, which is that as you get older sexual intercourse is to be less frequent, more for physiological reasons than anything else, so they have this idea in their head that as they get older they shouldn't be doing it as often, and I often find that patients will come, particularly if they have gone into a new relationship perhaps a second marriage or something like that, asking for permission, is it alright to feel like this? For them, it's being deviant from the accepted norm or of that norm which they have been fed, so I think they have this expectation in which case there's equally an ignorance of reality, I guess.

(male GP, aged 40–49)

One participant's account of 'permission-granting' warrants further attention as it departed from this popular view that GPs could help older people resist societal stereotypes of an 'asexual old age'. On the contrary, this participant felt that, as a result of the wider sexualization of society, older people were under increasing pressure to adopt 'younger' lifestyles, including to remain sexually active:

I also think older people have lost something of what it means to be older and to just appreciate and be content in that and are, in their effort, perhaps to feel valued and accepted in society, are trying to look, feel and do younger things, instead of enjoying a very companionable relationship, which may actually be an awful lot stronger in relationship terms, than some younger relationship which is based on sex. They are now defining themselves more by what would be natural in a younger relationship and are seeking to model that. So I think, yes, now I'm only seeing a relatively small number of people coming in but what I sense is behind it is older people looking to younger lifestyles and younger activities and thinking they ought to emulate it.

(male GP, aged 40–49)

Within this context he saw his role not as a permission granter to remain sexually active, but rather as legitimizing the choices of older people who did not want to have a sexual relationship, but felt 'pressured' into this:

I just want to check out they are not just falling foul of the marketing on sex really, and what does their spouse or partner feel about it? Are they agreeable to that or is it for some reason the guy has been watching TV films and now feels that he really ought to be a male or something and actually getting back into all that after a break can jeopardize his relationship, at least if he hasn't talked it through. So, yes, is it a restart after quite a period of break? Is it a new relationship? With older people who are much more canny and aware of non-sexual relationship issues, I'll seek to strengthen the companionship and friendship mode of the relationship.

(male GP, aged 40–49)

This quotation again indicates that participants saw their roles as extending beyond the strictly medical management of sexual health problems to assume a wider responsibility for the patient's overall relationship. The notion of 'permission granting' is therefore not only an interesting example of how medicine 'regulates' and defines sexuality (Foucault 1979), but also indicates the complexity of addressing sexual health for medical practitioners.

Raising sexual issues with older people

While participants acknowledged the importance of sexuality in later life in theory, they reported that they would be more likely to raise sexual issues with younger patients than older patients and, indeed, did so very infrequently with older patients. They also reported that older patients were unlikely to raise sexual issues proactively with them, with many participants reporting anecdotes of when this had happened and their resultant 'surprise'. The age bias in raising sexual issues with patients was particularly apparent within GP discussions of diagnosing conditions such as depression where sexual interest may be affected, as well as accounts of prescribing medications with known effects on sexual health. The account of the following GP participant was typical:

R: Is it quite standard for you to raise that [ED] if that's one of the key side-effects.

GP: Around diabetes and blood pressure ... say a man in his forties, I might warn him and say, 'this can have an effect on your sex drive', some men find it causes problems. I might not mention it to a man in his seventies so maybe that's a barrier that I'm putting up whereas I would assume a man in his forties would be married and sexually active but I might not assume a man of 70 was and I wouldn't know whether to bring it up unless he did. Same with the women really. So I suppose age is a big barrier, you do treat people differently in terms of their sexual health, I think.

(female GP, aged 40–49)

Similarly, most practice nurse participants commented that the age of the patient altered their approach in consultations and that more 'distinct cues' were required if they were to raise sexual issues with older patients:

I suppose you would realistically be more likely to raise issues like that with a 30-year-old than an 80-year-old, yeah. I mean, sometimes you might do but I would look for more distinct cues from them, in an older person, before I raise the issues, whereas in a younger person, I might be more inclined to raise the issues myself, I think, yeah, I think that's probably true.

(practice nurse, aged 40–49)

Interestingly, one of these cues could be the manner and appearance of the older patient, contrasting the 'sprightly' with the 'frail'. These judgements were less clinical than social:

You can tell with certain individuals, you shouldn't presume but some people are fitter than me at 70 and look happy about themselves, and how they keep, so [I] suppose you would, then, think, well, yes, these people are fit and healthy and probably do, you know. I suppose you tag it with health, don't you?

(practice nurse, aged 40–49)

This finding indicates that the connection between sex and health within contemporary society (Hawkes 1996) and discussed as a key contributory factor to the stereotype of the 'asexual old age' in Chapter 1, also influences health professional attitudes.

Barriers to discussing sexual health with older patients

Many of the barriers to discussing sexual issues with older patients were actually common to patients of all ages. These barriers are reported elsewhere (Gott et al. 2004) and are described well by participants' use of the term 'can of worms' to express their beliefs that sexually-related issues are highly problematic within primary care because of their sensitivity, complexity and constraints of time and expertise. Particular barriers were identified to discussing sexual health with patients of the opposite gender, patients from black and ethnic minority groups and non-heterosexual patients.

This section will focus upon those barriers that were felt to be specific to discussing sex with older patients including: attitudes towards later life sexuality; sexual health priorities not perceived as relevant to older people; communication and training issues; and sex being perceived as 'private' for older people.

Attitudes towards later life sexuality and sexual health

Overall, participants identified that many of the beliefs they held about sexuality in later life were based upon supposition rather than 'fact' or experience. Such beliefs were often acknowledged to be deep-rooted and, as such, influence the management of older people's sexual health concerns in a subconscious way. Participants were aware, for example, that their decisions to discuss 'safe sex' with patients of different ages were often based on stereotyped views of later life relationships:

> Int: I wonder … , whether you ever talked about safe sex with older people?
>
> GP: No …
>
> Int: Do you with younger people?
>
> GP: Mainly young people on the pill, to say it doesn't provide a physical barrier.
>
> Int: Why do you think that is, that you don't …?
>
> GP: Because I tend to think they are in monogamous, heterosexual relationships, because that's my stereotype for the older person.
>
> (male GP, aged 50–59)

Similarly, participants acknowledged that they also tended to think of sex as less relevant and less important to older people and that this attitude could form a barrier to raising sexual issues with this patient cohort. However, again these attitudes were based upon their own preconceptions:

> You know when you're young, it's all about, isn't it, kissing, canoodling and it's fun, and it's the whole ball game of meeting somebody, falling in love, out of love, in love. But I think for the majority of older people, once they're settled, their family growing up, it's more stable, it's just easy, isn't it, they are not looking for anybody any more, they are not striving for anything, it becomes the comfortable chair.
>
> (practice nurse, aged 50–59)

There was also awareness among a minority of participants that it was important not to talk about 'older people' as if age was a unifying force. Indeed, media and society images of sex in older age were contrasted with personal experience and that presented to them in consultations.

> I think it varies very much from person to person, I don't think you can generalize at all. I mean, the general view is, erm, that sex is something that, erm, or sexual enjoyment and experience is something that wanes with age but that's not really part of my own personal experience or the experience of some of the people that I am dealing with, and I think sexual issues are just as important for older people to be able to talk about as it is with younger people. The media, it's all young, beautiful people, but I have a lot of retired people [who] are still sexually active, you know, and are happy with that. A lot of it is to do with how people feel about themselves and it's sort of about relationships as well.
>
> (practice nurse, aged 40–49)

However, overall, a lack of recognition of the heterogeneity of later life was identified and stereotypes of older people's sexual behaviours and attitudes did form a significant barrier to talking about sex with this age group for most participants. These attitudes and behaviours were underpinned by wider societal attitudes towards ageing and sexuality, as well as personal ethical and religious beliefs. For example, within this context some participants discussed the link between sex and procreation:

> Certainly, from my upbringing as a Catholic, sex was for the production of children so as soon as you stop producing children, what on earth do you want to do it for, and we have got to move away from that and say, actually, it's an enjoyable activity that is no different really to going and watching films in terms of the pleasure it brings.
>
> (male GP, aged 30–39)

Finally, for a minority of participants the discomfort that many felt in discussing sex with older patients was heightened by personal beliefs that later life sexuality was 'revolting' or 'disgusting'. One participant in particular expressed her beliefs in this way:

> GP: The older they are the worse it is, for me.
> Int: So if it was an 85-year-old ...
> GP: I would find that quite unpalatable ... Yes I hope that I don't display my repugnance [laughs] when the 85-year-old turns up for his Viagra, I hope that if they need referring I refer them appropriately, but I certainly never go delving for information in that department with the old ones.
>
> (female GP, aged 50–59)

However, this was an extreme viewpoint not shared by the remaining participants.

Sexual health priorities within primary care not perceived as relevant to older people

Overall, and as noted above, participants' attitudes towards sexual health priorities within primary care reflected national policy, focusing as they did on providing contraceptive advice and preventing and managing STIs. In relation to contraceptive advice, an identified implication of not holding such discussions with post-menopausal women was that it resulted in a lack of clear opportunities to raise sexual health issues with this patient group. The other significant priority within primary care, namely STI prevention and management, was also not seen as relevant to middle-aged and older patients. This was apparent in accounts such as this, where STIs are framed very much as a younger persons issue:

> we're doing a bit of a research area on the *younger end* and offering opportunistically when they come for pill checks, etcetera, making them aware of chlamydia and sexually transmitted diseases and offering that service for swabs, so we have had a few that have come of their own accord for that so it can be anything from contraception, sexual contact, infection, morning-after pill or relationship problems, either of sexual or psychosexual nature.
>
> (practice nurse, aged 30–39)

Indeed, many participants reacted with amusement when asked if they ever talked about 'safe sex' with their older patients as in this example where the participant was asked if he ever discussed such issues with older patients who form new partnerships in later life:

> Int: Do you ever talk to older people about safe sex?
> GP: No [laughs] because usually the context seems totally inappropriate. They are usually people that they have known for twenty or thirty years as close friends, and have probably harboured feelings about. That part of society, they just wouldn't have had affairs, that we know about. They're not going out cruising [laughs], it's usually a very personal thing, so no, no.
>
> (male GP, aged 40–49)

This situation was seen to be even more complex to address with older people in long-term relationships:

> I think it's difficult if you think somebody has got a sexually transmitted infection and you get it wrong and that can cause deep offence, and that's another thing that stops you thinking about sexually transmitted diseases in elderly people and maybe not doing all the swabs, because it's very hard talking to someone who is in a relationship, who you know has been in a relationship for 30 years, 'could there be a chance of any STI?' You know it hits at the heart of our relationships and ourselves, so yes I have caused offence so I don't take any risks with that.
>
> (female GP: aged 40–49)

This participant also related the fact that she did not discuss safe sex with older patients to the age distribution of STI prevalence:

> GP: You're talking about risks and you don't want to get neurotic 80-year-olds worrying about HIV or hepatitis B, you know, if they are having sex every now and then, which is probably mostly what it is. So I think there is a caring behind it and also being sensible. It is more significant if somebody of 20 becomes HIV or hepatitis B positive and it's more likely to happen because it's more prevalent in those age groups, so the risk gets less as you get older. It always feels like it might be a bit politically correct to talk to 60, 70 or 80 year olds about these things, but actually is it really right for the person?
> Int: But what about, say, forties and fifties?
> GP: Yes, it gets to be a gradation really.
> Int: Would you talk to a person in their forties or fifties about safe sex?
> GP: Probably not.
>
> (female GP, aged 40–49)

This extract also exemplifies how participants tended to subsume a very large age range of people within the category of 'older people', and rarely acknowledged later life heterogeneity.

Communication and training issues

Overall, participants identified that they found it a lot more 'difficult' to discuss sexual issues with older patients than younger patients. A key reason for this discomfort was seen to be the fact that sex was not a topic they would normally discuss with people of this age group, for example, their parents:

> I'm 50, so my upbringing was extremely Victorian and I don't think I have ever discussed anything to do with sex with my mother and certainly not my dad, you know you just didn't do it ... So, yes, I have got lots of hang-ups, lots and lots.
>
> (female GP, aged 50–59)

Practice nurses also identified that the age and gender gap between them and their older male patients meant that issues such as erectile dysfunction were raised with them infrequently:

> They tend to go to the male doctors, I've found, because I think, especially the older end, because they think 'oh God' you know 'a young nurse, [lowers voice] I don't want to talk about anything like that' and they go and see the male doctor.
>
> (practice nurse, aged 30–39)

These communication difficulties were not addressed in participants' training, which overall was felt to be inadequate in relation to sexual health: 'In some ways you talk to younger people because you are trained to do that and you do what you are trained to do. Nobody has ever trained me to talk to older people' (female GP, aged 50–59). Furthermore, participants who were involved in medical student teaching at the present time identified that this was still not a topic that was routinely addressed:

> The way we teach them [medical students], the scenarios we use are very much age-related, in fact the examination question is about a 30-year-old. I think it would be fascinating to write one based on a 60-year-old and see what they say, because I think it would definitely add another barrier, especially if their perception is that people stop having sex at the age of 50 or something like that.
>
> (male GP, aged 30–39)

However, although some participants would welcome training opportunities in relation to later life sexual health management, all acknowledged that they had limited time and resources to participate in such training, even if suitable opportunities were available.

Sex as 'private' for older people and the risk of causing offence

One strong theme to emerge from the findings related to participants' perceptions that older people view sex and sexual health issues as more 'private' and personal than younger people. This was related to the perceived impact of growing up in a time when sex was not discussed as openly as it is today:

> I think the older generations, because of the way that they were brought up, it is more difficult for quite a few of those, because it's difficult to get out of the way you were brought up, because if you were very open at home and people talked about those thing, then you're going to be open to other areas. If you have a problem you come and talk about it. But if things were never talked about and it was always hush, hush and don't talk about that, then it must be difficult to get out of that.
>
> (practice nurse, aged 40–49)

These beliefs that sex was 'private' for older people were identified as translating into clinical practice, for example, a GP participant reported that: 'I wouldn't dream of saying we do a sexual health clinic for the over-40s on a Tuesday afternoon, which you can do for the under-20s. It's a much more personal private thing I think' (female GP, aged 50–59).

There were also concerns expressed that people of this age see these 'private' issues as not being legitimate topics for discussion within a health care setting. As a result, participants identified that they had to think carefully before initiating discussions of sexual issues with older patients because they didn't want patients to think that they were 'prying into something that's not my business' (male GP, aged 40–49). Raising such issues inappropriately was identified as having the potential to cause offence. This was identified as a particular concern by GP participants, who felt it could cause significant damage to the patient–doctor relationship and, in particular, compromise the GP's professional competence in the eyes of the patient.

> Int: I'm interested in the idea of offending someone – does it matter if you offend someone?
> GP: Yes, it does, very much so ... if you mention something like that, 'You know, this will affect your sex life' to an older woman who sort of hasn't slept with her husband for years and years, you know she might be quite sensitive to the fact that she hasn't slept with her husband for years and years and might be quite upset if you said that and I think that's going to break down your doctor–patient relationship if somebody says that. You have to be very careful sometimes or you'll never see them again, they'll go to see somebody else ... I think if somebody starts making assumptions about your sex life, which are not true, then, yes they would get very offended. That's the danger [laughs].
>
> (female GP, aged 30–39)

Interestingly, however, when participants were asked to give examples of when they had offended an older person by raising a sexual issue within an inappropriate context, very few could recall an occasion when this had happened:

> I think sometimes as well people would be a bit affronted, you know, older people, I suppose, they haven't always thought of sex like that in the way that younger people do and would be far more open about talking about infections and stuff like that, for older people that's harder and maybe you pick up on their awkwardness with it as well and you don't, you don't, go down that path so much ... I'm trying to think of an example, I'm sure something has happened similar to that (pauses). I can't think of anything.
>
> (practice nurse, aged 40–49)

Such quotations indicate that decisions by GPs and practice nurses to raise sexual issues in consultations are influenced more by their perception that sex is difficult and potentially offensive to address, rather than direct personal experience supporting this belief. This situation was particularly marked in relation to older people due to a tendency to view later life sexuality in a stereotyped and homogenous way, as noted previously in this discussion. Training using 'experiential methods to recognize each individual's unique experience of sex and sexuality' has been recommended as being appropriate to break down stereotypes of particular patient groups (Curtis et al. 1995: 113). However, as discussed below, the context of limited time and financial resources within primary care are likely to prove an impediment to the development and uptake of training in this area.

Summary of findings

To summarize, this study identified that:

- Sexual health was equated with sexual risk-taking and younger people.
- Participants were aware that they could 'give permission' for older people to discuss sex in consultations, although in reality this occurred infrequently. There was also evidence that older people may ask GPs for moral guidance on the appropriateness of being sexually active in later life.
- Participants reported that they were much less likely to initiate discussions of sexual issues with older patients than younger patients and required more distinct (often social) cues to do so.
- Specific barriers to discussing sex with older patients included: beliefs about sexuality in later life (based on stereotypes rather than direct experience of individual patients); sexual health priorities not perceived as relevant to older people; sexual health training having been in relation to younger people; and sex being perceived as 'private' for older people.

Conclusion

As discussed in the introduction to this chapter, an increasingly significant role has been defined for health professionals in sexual health management and, in particular, in later life sexual health management. Kessel, for example, states that: 'Professionals should advise that sex is good for you and orgasm achieved by masturbation may relieve anxiety and promote well-being' (2001: 122). Similarly, Wallace (2003: 53) argues: 'Despite the barriers, the continuing sexual needs of the elderly must be addressed [by professionals] with the same priority as nutrition, hydration, and other well-accepted needs.' However, findings from the above study indicate that this (arguably inappropriate) rhetoric is very far from the reality. In practice, sex is neither prioritized, nor even frequently discussed with older patients. The issue of the limits to professional responsibility for later life sexual health management will be addressed at the end of this section.

In order to address the gap between current recommendations and clinical reality, participants in the above study were asked to reflect on ways in which they could be better prepared to meet the sexual health needs of older patients. Three key recommendations were made. First, a need for training was identified, although it was felt that this would only be taken up by a minority of professionals and was difficult to pursue given time constraints. Nevertheless, such training should be made available for those who desire it. Second, GP participants in particular recommended an expanded role for nursing in sexual health management. However, while many nurse participants were interested in adopting such a role, they identified gender as a key barrier to so doing. Indeed, a patient preference for same-sex consultations was seen to limit the opportunities to discuss sexual issues with older men given that virtually all practice nurses in the UK are female (Richards, chair RCN Practice Nurse Association, personal communication), although it could be a possibility in relation to older women. Finally, it was suggested that providing information targeted at older patients and highlighting that sexual health is an appropriate topic to be discussed with a health care professional could empower older people themselves to present with sexual health concerns. While this certainly seems a very good idea, sexual health literature tends to be focused very much on STI prevention and targeted at younger people. Therefore, more appropriate literature needs to be produced which may indeed help older patients discuss sexually related concerns in this way.

The study findings also highlight key situations where sexual health issues should be raised by health professionals working with older patients, but are not at the present time. For example, in the previous chapter, older men reported erectile dysfunction which they attributed to particular medications. However, because this had not been mentioned as a potential side-effect of the medication by a health professional, they did not feel it was an issue that would be taken seriously 'at their age'. The accounts of GPs and practice nurses presented in this chapter confirm that the sexual side-effects of diagnosed health conditions or prescribed medications are not raised proactively with older patients. However, older age should not be a factor in determining whether sexual health issues are raised in a patient consultation or not. Indeed, while the National Service Framework for older people may have said nothing about sexual health, it did stress the importance of ending age discrimination within UK health settings (DoH 2001a).

In a similar vein, professionals should not assume that older people are immune from contracting STIs. The data presented in Chapter 6 indicate that this is certainly not the case, with significant rates of STIs, including HIV and AIDS, having been diagnosed in this older age group. Moreover, we can expect rates of sexual risk-taking and related STIs to increase among older people over the coming years due to expected cohort changes in sexual attitudes and behaviours. However, this does not appear to have been acknowledged within either policy or practice where STIs are still seen as a concern only to younger people.

Overall, the myth of the 'asexual' older person who, if sexually active, must be so within the context of a mutually monogamous, heterosexual relationship still appears to underpin the attitudes and behaviours of most health professionals. This was very apparent in the accounts of the participants in the study above, where attitudes towards later life sexual health management were determined by stereotypes of older people, rather than direct experience with older patients. For example, 'causing offence' was seen as a key reason not to discuss sex with older patients – however, as noted above, very few participants could give an example of when they had done so. Therefore, a key recommendation for health professionals arising from this research must be not to make assumptions about a person's sexual attitudes and behaviours on the basis of age. Indeed, evidence has been presented indicating that older people welcome sexual issues being raised with them in an appropriate context. The professional challenge is to ensure this happens.

Finally, it is important to return to the published recommendations about later life sexual health management previously mentioned in these discussions. First, these can be argued to afford an undue importance to sex, for example, equating sexual pleasure with adequate nutrition and hydration seems highly misguided. As argued in Chapter 2, not having sex may make you unhappy, but it does not make you sick, let alone have the potential to kill you (Gannon 1999). In addition, the GP and practice nurse accounts presented above indicate that recommendations to promote masturbation and the importance of orgasms with older patients (Kessel 2001) are not only inappropriate, but also so far from professional's day-to-day clinical practice as to be completely unrealistic. Moreover, they invoke thoughts about when professional responsibility for meeting the sexual health needs of older patients ends.

This is an issue which has already been subject to extensive, heated debate within the nursing press in relation to nurse responsibility for addressing the sexual concerns of people with disabilities. In Canada, for example, nurses were sacked for refusing to adhere to a new 'sexual assistance' policy where nurses were expected to assume an active role in their disabled clients' sex lives, for example, through putting on a condom or helping them watch pornographic videos. This case sparked controversy among UK nurses. In particular, the call from Gill Aylott, a member of the Royal College of Nursing Learning Disabilities Forum (Coombes 1998) for a similar policy in the UK and, in particular, her view that nurses should help clients masturbate, was met with indignation. One nursing student, for example, wrote that not only does this approach imply that disabled people need the help of qualified professionals to be sexually fulfilled, but also that she was not relishing 'the prospect of completing my four-year nursing degree in order to become one of the lowest paid prostitutes in the country' (Gibson 1998: 12).

While the professional literature aimed at those working with older people has not entered into debates such as this as yet, it seems this may only be a matter of time. Indeed, (ageist) claims that older people need professional help to be sexually satisfied is certainly a recurrent theme within the medical and nursing literature. It seems highly appropriate therefore to begin considering where health professional responsibility for older people's sexual health ends. It is helpful within this context to draw a line between advice and advocacy. Indeed, there has been a tendency within the sexuality and ageing literature to call for health professionals to promote sex as an important contributory factor to overall well-being among older people. Hajjar and Kamel (2003: 578), for example, argue that:

> Despite the known benefits of continued sexual activity on physical, mental, and emotional health, the nursing home resident continues to

be sexually invisible. There are so few opportunities where the quality of life can be enhanced so greatly by so basic interventions.

They go on to outline how professionals working with this group of older people can encourage them to be sexually active and fulfilled. However, not only does writing such as this contribute to the idea that older people cannot do anything to maximize their own sexual satisfaction, but it also can be argued to be advocating sexual activity inappropriately. Promoting sex is not the same as promoting healthy eating or regular exercise. This needs to be acknowledged if workable recommendations regarding professional involvement in later life sexual health management are to be produced.

To conclude, this chapter has identified that sex is a very difficult topic to discuss within patient consultations and, in particular, sexual health issues are rarely discussed in consultations with older people. It has been argued that recommendations for professional involvement in this area need to be more realistic than those published to date in the sexuality and ageing literature and, in particular, should acknowledge limits of time, experience and expertise. However, ultimately it is crucial that older age ceases to be perceived as a major determinant of sexual health management.

Acknowledgements

Extracts from this chapter are based on the following paper and are reproduced with the permission of Elsevier: Gott, M., Hinchliff, S. and Galena, E. (2004) A qualitative study to explore GP attitudes to discussing sexual health issues with older people, *Social Science and Medicine*, 58(11): 2093–103.

The study was funded by an unrestricted educational grant from Pfizer Ltd. However, the study protocol and all publications arising from it are *solely* the work of the authors.

I would like to thank Sharron Hinchliff, Elisabeth Galena and Helen Elford for their invaluable contribution to this research, and all study participants for their time.

9

Conclusion

My task in this book has been to critically examine the relationship between sexuality, sexual health and ageing within a wider context than has previously been adopted. In particular, I have argued for a need to situate such discussions within a theoretical framework which challenges us to explore, both what we mean by concepts such as 'sexuality' and 'old age', and how we have arrived at such understandings. On embarking upon this exploration it becomes apparent that there is a real need to move away from viewing these as 'natural' and fixed by biology. So doing opens up numerous possibilities. Crucially, it indicates that the 'myth of the asexual old age' has not emerged because we do not have sufficient proof that older people have sex (as has typically been assumed within the sexuality and ageing literature). Rather, in considering societal norms that set boundaries around how someone comes to be defined as 'sexual', the incompatibility between old age and sexuality becomes highly evident. Sexuality is all that old age is not: healthy, beautiful, powerful and, crucially, youthful.

Taking a similar approach led to a critique of the emerging stereotype of what I have termed the 'sexy oldie'. While this new way of conceptualizing sexuality and ageing may initially appear (and has been argued to be) liberating for older people, when examined in more detail, it can be seen as anything but. Adults of all ages are left with little choice but to be 'sexual' to remain socially engaged. So doing is defined in youthful terms – looking young (by whatever means) is crucial, as is engaging in the gold standard of sexual expression, namely sexual intercourse. Moreover, when the factors underpinning this new view of ageing sexuality are examined, issues of profit and power come to be of central concern.

A further key aim of these discussions has been to add the voices of older people themselves to debates on later life sexuality. Findings were reported from a qualitative study which identified the value (and feasibility) of talking to older people about sexual issues. More work in this vein is needed to enable research to move away from an obsession with identifying how often older people 'do it' and conceptualize sexuality as part of the totality of later life experience.

I have been keen to stress the importance of recognizing the diversity of later life experience. While this is certainly not a new idea within gerontology, writings about sexuality within the context of ageing have tended to assume a (false) commonality by age. It has been argued that differences of gender, socio-economic class, age cohort, geography, sexual orientation and ethnicity (to name but a few) must assume centrality in discussions of later life sexual attitudes and experiences. We know little about how such differences shape older people's beliefs about sexuality and this warrants further attention.

While the ever-tightening bond between sexuality and medicine was critiqued, the tendency to view sexuality from a 'health' perspective is certainly set to continue. Therefore, a need to consider sexual health within the context of ageing was identified. While there is evidence that older people experience sexual problems (albeit limited by the exclusion of older people from sexual health research), later life sexual health needs are often neither acknowledged nor addressed within sexual health policy and practice. However, using (older) age as a criterion for determining which individuals should be asked about their sexual health needs goes against NHS principles aimed at rooting out age discrimination in health service delivery (Department of Health 2001a).

To conclude, it is worth returning to consider the exalted position afforded to sexuality within contemporary Western society. Indeed, while sexuality ties us up in knots with its complexities and the powerful emotions it provokes, its importance for us both individually and collectively is unprecedented. Indeed, at this point in time, and within the context of these discussions as a whole, Foucault's words seem more apt than ever:

> Over the centuries it [sex] has become more important than our soul, more important almost than our life ... Perhaps one day people will wonder at this. They will not be able to understand how a civilization so intent on developing enormous instruments of production and destruction found the time and infinite patience to inquire so anxiously concerning the actual state of sex.
>
> (1979: 156–8)

References

Addley, E. (2001) If you weren't sick, you would think it was a five-star hotel, *The Guardian*. http://society.guardian.co.uk/health/story/0,7890,441436,00.html (accessed 25 May 2004).

Adler, M.W. (1997) Sexual health: a health of the nation failure, *British Medical Journal*, 314: 1743–47.

Adler, M.W. (1998) Sexual health: is an important part of people's lives and doctors need to understand its variety, *British Medical Journal*, 317: 1470.

Age Concern (1995) *A Crisis of Silence*, 2nd edn. London: Age Concern.

Age Concern (2002) *Opening Doors Conference: Summary Report*. London: Age Concern.

Ahmadi, N. (2003) Rocking sexualities: Iranian migrants' views on sexuality, *Archives of Sexual Behaviour*, 32(4): 317–26.

American Academy of Anti-Aging Medicine. http://www.worldhealth.net/index.php?p=77 (accessed 24 Oct. 2003).

American Psychiatric Association (1994) *Diagnostic and Statistical Manual of Mental Disorders*, 4th edn. Washington, DC: American Psychiatric Association.

Aral, S.O. and Wasserheit, J.N. (1997) STD-related health care seeking and health service delivery, in K.K. Holmes, P.A. Mardh, S.M. Lemon, W.E. Stamm and J.N. Piot (eds) *Sexually Transmitted Diseases*, 3rd edn. New York: McGraw-Hill.

Arber, S., Davidson, K. and Ginn, J. (eds) (2003) *Gender and Ageing: Changing Roles and Relationships*. Buckingham: Open University Press.

Arber, S.L. and Ginn, J. (eds) (1995) *Connecting Gender and Ageing: A Sociological Approach*. Buckingham: Open University Press.

Archibald, C. (1998) Sexuality, dementia and residential care: managers' report and response, *Health and Social Care in the Community*, 6(2): 95–101.

Archibald, C. (2002) Sexuality and dementia in residential care – whose responsibility?, *Sexual and Relationship Therapy*, 17(3) 301–10.

Askham, J. and Stewart, E. (1995) *Breaking the Silence*. London: Age Concern England.

Bacon, C.G., Mittleman, M.A., Kawachi, I., Giovannucci, E., Glasser, D.B. and Rimm, E.B. (2003) Sexual function in men older than 50 years of age: results from the health professionals' follow-up study, *Annals of Internal Medicine*, 139(3): 161–8.

Bancroft, J. (1983) *Human Sexuality and its Problems*. Edinburgh: Churchill Livingstone.

Bancroft, J. (1998) Alfred Kinsey's work 50 years later, in A.C. Kinsey, W.B. Pomeroy, E.E. Martin and P.H. Gebhard (eds) *Sexual Behaviour in the Human Female*. New York: WB Sanders, Reprinted.

Bankhead, C. (1997) New field could open up for urologists: Female sexual dysfunction, *Urology Times*, 25(1): 39.

Baraniak, C. et al. (2002) Re: Can nurse practitioners provide equivalent care to GPs, letter to editor, *British Medical Journal*, 324(7341): 819.

Barrow, G.M. (1992) *Aging, the Individual and Society*. New York: West Publishing Company.

Bennett, K.C. and Thompson, N.L. (1990) Accelerated aging and male homosexuality: Australian evidence in a continuing debate, in J.A. Lee (ed.) *Gay Midlife and Maturity*. Binghampton and London: Harrington Park Press.

Berman, J.R. and Bassuk, J. (2002) Physiology and pathophysiology of female sexual function and dysfunction, *World Journal of Urology*, 20(2): 111–18.

Biggs, S. (1999) *The Mature Imagination: Dynamics of Identity in Midlife and Beyond*. Buckingham: Open University Press.

Birch, S. (2001) Out of the closet, *The Guardian*. http://society.guardian.co.uk/society guardian/story/O,,526672,OO.html (accessed 9 October 2004).

Blaikie, A. (1999) *Ageing and Popular Culture*. Cambridge: Cambridge University Press.

Blakemore, K., Boneham, M. and Gearing, B. (1993) *Age, Race and Ethnicity: A Comparative Approach*. Buckingham: Open University Press.

Bland, R. (1999) Independence, privacy and risk: two contrasting approaches to residential care for older people, *Ageing and Society*, 19(5): 539–60.

Bortz, W.M., Wallace, D.H. and Wiley, D. (1999) Sexual function in 1202 aging males: differentiating aspects, *Journal of Gerontology*, 54(5): 237–41.

Braun, M., Wassmer, G., Klotz, T., Reifenrath, B., Mathers, M. and Engelmann, U. (2000) Epidemiology of erectile dysfunction: results of the 'Cologne Male Survey', *International Journal of Impotence Research*, 12(6): 305–11.

Brecher, E.M. (1984) *Love, Sex and Aging: Consumer Union Report*. Boston: Little Brown and Co.

Bretschneider, J.G. and McCoy, N.L. (1988) Sexual interest and behavior in healthy 80 to 102 year olds, *Archives of Sexual Behaviour*, 17(2): 109–29.

Bristow, J. (1997) *Sexuality*. London and New York: Routledge.

Brogan, M. (1996) The sexual needs of elderly people: addressing the issue, *Nursing Standard*, 10(24): 42–5.

Brown, L. (1989) Is there sexual freedom for our aging population in long-term care institutions?, *Journal of Gerontological Social Work*, 13: 75–93.

Bullard-Poe, L., Powell, C. and Mulligan, T. (1994) The importance of intimacy to men living in a nursing home, *Archives of Sexual Behavior*, 23(2): 231–6.

Bullock, K. (2001) Healthy Family Systems? The changing role of grandparents in rural America, *Education and Ageing*, 16(2): 163–78.

Burns, A., Jacoby, R. and Levy, R. (1990) Psychiatric phenomena in Alzheimer's Disease, *British Journal of Psychiatry*, 157: 86–94.

Butler, R.N. and Lewis, M.I. (2002) *The New Love and Sex After 60*. New York: Ballantine Books.

Bytheway, B. (1995) *Ageism*. Buckingham and Philadelphia: Open University Press.

Catania, J.A., McDermott, L.J. and Pollack, L.M. (1986) Questionnaire response bias and face-to-face interview sample bias in sexuality research, *The Journal of Sex Research*, 22(1): 52–72.

Centers for Disease Control and Prevention HIV and AIDS – United States, 1981–2000. *MMWR* 2001: 50: 430–4.

Charmaz, K. (1983) Loss of self: a fundamental form of suffering in the chronically ill, *Sociology of Health and Illness*, 5(2): 168–95.

Clark, J.A., Bokhour, B.G., Inui, T.S., Silliman, R.A. and Talcott, J.A. (2003) Measuring patients' perceptions of the outcomes of treatment for early prostate cancer, *Medical Care*, 41(8): 923–36.

Cole, T.R. (1992) *The Journey of Life: A Cultural History of Aging in America*. Cambridge: Cambridge University Press.

Coombes, R. (1998) Is this asking nurses to go too far?, *Nursing Times*, 94(16): 12–13, 22–8.

Cotrell, V. and Shultz, R. (1993) The perspective of the patient with Alzheimer's Disease: a neglected dimension of dementia research, *The Gerontologist*, 33: 205–11.

Cranston, R.D. and Thin, R.N. (1998) Sexually transmitted infection in the elderly, *Sexually Transmitted Infections*, 74: 314–15.

Cunningham-Burley, S., Allbutt, H., Garraway, W.M., Lee, A.J. and Russell, E.B.A.W. (1996) Perceptions of urinary symptoms and health-care-seeking behaviour amongst men aged 40–79 years, *British Journal of General Practice*, 46: 349–52.

Curtis, H., Hoolaghan, T. and Jewitt, C. (1995) *Sexual Health Promotion in General Practice*. Oxford: Radcliffe Medical.

Daker-White, G. and Donovan, J. (2002) Sexual satisfaction, quality of life and the transaction of intimacy in hospital patients' accounts of their (hetero)sexual relationships, *Sociology of Health and Illness*, 24(1): 89–113.

Davidson, K. (2000) What we want: older widows and widowers speak for themselves, *Journal of the British Association of Social Workers*, 12(1): 45–54.

Deacon, S., Minichiello, V. and Plummer, D. (1995) Sexuality and older people: revisiting the assumptions, *Educational Gerontology*, 21: 497–513.

Dean, M. (2003) End pensioner poverty, *The Guardian*. http://society. guardian.co.uk/ socialexclusion/comment/0,11499,1108237,00.html (accessed 17 Dec. 2003).

deGraft Agyarko, R., Madzingira, N., Mupedziswa, R., Mujuru, N., Kanyowa, L. and Matorofa, J. (2002) *Impact of AIDS on Older People in Africa: Zimbabwe Case Study*. Geneva: WHO.

Department of Health (2001a) *National Service Framework for Older People*. London: HMSO.

Department of Health (2001b) *National Sexual Health Strategy*. London: HMSO.

Department of Health, England and Wales General and Personal Medical Services Statistics (2003). Available online: http://www.publications.doh.gov.uk/public/ gpcensus2003tab4.xls (accessed 16 June 2004).

Derouesne, C., Guigot, J., Chermat, V., Winchester, N. and Lacomblez, L. (1996) Sexual behavioural changes in Alzheimer Disease, *Alzheimer Disease and Associated Disorders*, 10(2): 86–92.

Dinnerstein, L. and Weitz, R. (1998) Jane Fonda, Barbara Bush, and other aging bodies: femininity and the limits of resistance, in R. Weitz (ed.) *The Politics of Women's Bodies*. New York and Oxford: Oxford University Press, pp. 198–204.

Diokono, A.C., Brown, M.B. and Herzog, A.R. (1990) Sexual function in the elderly, *Archives of Internal Medicine*, 150(1): 197–200.

Dolcini, M.M., Catania, J.A., Stall, D.A. and Pollack, L. (2003) The HIV epidemic among older men who have sex with men, *Journal of Acquired Immune Deficiency Syndromes*, 33(2): S115–S121.

Duddle, C.M. (1982) Influences on sex – elderly; psychological and physiological and social stigma, *Geriatric Medicine*, 65–8.

Duffy, L.M. (1998) Lovers, loners, and lifers: sexuality and the older adult, *Geriatrics*, 53(1): 66–9.

Duncan, B., Hart, G., Scoular, A. and Bigrigg, A. (2001) Qualitative analysis of psychosocial impact of diagnosis of chlamydia trachomatis: implications for screening, *British Medical Journal*, 322(7280): 195–9.

Duncan, B., Sheeran, P., Spencer, C.P. et al. (1995) Delay in seeking treatment for STD: an application of protection motivation theory in a clinical setting, *Proc. BPS*, 3: 51.

Duncombe, J. and Marsden, D. (1996) Whose orgasm is it anyway? 'Sex work' in long term heterosexual couples relationships, in W. Weeks and J. Holland (eds) *Sexual Cultures, Communities, Values and Intimacy*. Basingstoke and London: Macmillan Press.

Dunn, K.M., Croft, P.R. and Hackett, G.I. (1998) Sexual problems: a study of the prevalence and need for health care in the general population, *Family Practice*, 15: 519–24.

Dunn, K.M., Croft, P.R. and Hackett, G.I. (1999) Association of sexual problems with social, psychological, and physical problems in men and women: a cross sectional population survey, *Journal of Epidemiology and Community Health*, 53(3): 144–8.

Edwards, D.J. (2003) Sex and intimacy in the nursing home, *Nursing Homes*. http://www.nursinghomesmagazine.com/Past_Issues.htm (accessed 13 Feb. 2004).

El-Sadr, W. and Gettler, J. (1995) Unrecognized human immunodeficiency virus infection in the elderly, *Archives of Internal Medicine*, 155: 184–6.

Ellis, H. (1933) *Psychology of Sex*. London: William Heinemann.

Ellison, C. (2000) Women's Sexualities: Generations of women share intimate secrets of sexual self-acceptance. Oakland, CA: New Harbinger.

Enzil, P., Mathieu, C., Vanderscheuren, D. and Demyttenaere, K. (1998) Diabetes Mellitus and female sexuality: a review of 25 years' research, *Diabetic Medicine*, 15: 809–15.

Estes, C.L. (1979) *The Aging Enterprise*. San Francisco: Jossey-Bass.

Estes, C.L. (1991) The new political economy of aging: introduction and critique, in M. Minkler and C. Estes (eds) *Critical Perspectives on Aging*. Amityville, NY: Baywood Publishing Company Inc.

Estes, C.L. and Binney, E.A. (1991) The biomedicalization of aging: dangers and dilemmas, in M. Minkler and C. Estes (eds) *Critical Perspectives on Aging: The Political and Moral Economy of Growing Old*. Amityville, NY: Baywood Publishing Company Inc.

Featherstone, M. (1991) *Consumer Culture and Postmodernism*. London: Sage.

Featherstone, M. and Hepworth, M. (1990) Images of ageing, in J. Bond and P. Coleman (eds) *Ageing in Society: An Introduction to Social Gerontology*. London: Sage.

Featherstone, M. and Wernick, A. (1995) *Images of Aging: Cultural Representations of Later Life*. London and New York: Routledge.

Feldman, H.A. et al. (1994) Impotence and its medical and psychosocial correlates: results of the Massachusetts Male Aging Study, *Journal of Urology*, 151: 54–61.

Flowers, P., Duncan, B. and Knussen, C. (2003) Reappraising HIV testing: an exploration of the psychosocial costs and benefits associated with learning one's HIV status in a purposive sample of Scottish gay men, *British Journal of Health Psychology*, 8: 179–94.

Ford, P. (1998) Sexuality and sexual health, in J. Marr and B. Kershaw (eds) *Caring for Older People: Developing Specialist Practice*. London: Arnold.

Fortenberry, J.D. (1997) Health care seeking behaviors related to sexually transmitted diseases among adolescents, *American Journal of Public Health*, 87(3): 417–20.

Foucault, M. (1979) *The History of Sexuality:* Vol. 1, *The Will to Knowledge*. London: Allen Lane.

Foucault, M. (1985) *The History of Sexuality:* Vol. 2, *The Use of Pleasure*. New York: Random House.

Foucault, M. (1986) *The History of Sexuality: The Care of the Self*, Vol. 3. New York: Random House.

Freud, S. (1977) *On Sexuality: Three Essays on the Theory of Sexuality and Other Works*. San Francisco: Pelican Books.

Friend, R.A. (1980) Gaying: adjustment and the older gay male, *Alternative Lifestyles*, 3: 231–48.

Friend, R.A. (1990) Older lesbian and gay people: a theory of successful aging, in J.A. Lee (ed.) *Gay Midlife and Maturity*. Binghampton and London: Harrington Park Press.

Furman, F.K. (1997) *Facing the Mirror: Older Women and Beauty Shop Culture*. New York and London: Routledge.

Gannon, L.R. (1999) *Women and Aging: Transcending the Myths*. London and New York: Routledge.

Gavey, N., McPhillips, K. and Braun, V. (1999) Interruptus coitus: heterosexuals accounting for intercourse, *Sexualities*, 2: 35–68.

George, K. and Weiler, S.J. (1981) Sexuality in middle and later life, *Archives of General Psychiatry*, 38: 919–23.

Gibson, T. (1992) *Love, Sex and Power in Later Life: A Libertarian Perspective*. London: Freedom Press.

Gibson, Y. (1998) A nursing model that has run amok. (Letter to editor), *Nursing Times*, 94(19): 12.

Giddens, A. (1992) *The Transformation of Intimacy: Sexuality, Love and Eroticism in Modern Societies*. Cambridge: Polity Press.

Gilleard, C. and Higgs, P. (2000) *Cultures of Ageing: Self, Citizen and the Body*. Harlow: Prentice Hall.

Gilmore, N. and Somerville, M.A. (1994) Stigmatization, scapegoating and discrimination in sexually transmitted diseases: overcoming 'them' and 'us', *Social Science and Medicine*, 39(9): 1339–58.

Glossman, H., Petrischor, G. and Bartsch, G. (1999) Molecular mechanisms of the effects of sildenafil (VIAGRA), *Experimental Gerontology*, 34(3): 305–18.

Goffman, E. (1961) *Asylums: Essays on the Social Situation of Mental Patients and Other Inmates*. New York: Anchor.

Goldstein, I. (2003) Womens' sexual woes get attention. http://www.cbsnews.com/stories/2004/05/03/eveningnews/main615320.shtml. (accessed 20 Feb. 2004).

Gordon, S.M. and Thompson, S. (1995) The changing epidemiology of human immunodeficiency virus infection in older persons, *Journal of the American Geriatrics Society*, 43(1): 7–9.

Gott, C.M., Ahmed, I., McKee, K.J., Morgan, K., Riley, V. and Rogstad, K.E. (1998) Characteristics of older patients attending GUM clinics, *Health Care in Later Life*, 3(4): 252–7.

Gott, C.M., Rogstad, K.E., Riley, V. and Ahmed-Jusuf, I. (1999) Delay in symptom presentation among a sample of older GUM clinic attenders, *International Journal of STD and AIDS*, 10: 43–6.

Gott, C.M., Rogstad, K.E., Riley, V., Ahmed-Jusuf, I. and Green, T. (2000) Exploring the sexual histories of older GUM clinic attenders, *International Journal of STD and AIDS*, 11(11). 714–18.

Gott, M. (2001) Sexual activity and risk-taking in later life, *Health and Social Care in the Community*, 9(2): 72–78.

Gott, M. and Hinchliff, S. (2002) An asexual old age: myth or reality?, in *Proceedings of the British Gerontology Society Annual Conference*. Birmingham: British Society of Gerontology.

Gott, M. and Hinchliff, S. (2003a) How important is sex in later life? The views of older people, *Social Science and Medicine*, 56(8): 1617–28.

Gott, M. and Hinchliff, S. (2003b) Barriers to seeking treatment for sexual problems in primary care: a qualitative study with older people, *Family Practice*, 20(6): 690–5.

Gott, M. and Hinchliff, S. (2003c) Sex and ageing: a gendered issue?, in S. Arber, K. Davidson and J. Ginn (eds) *Gender and Ageing: New Directions*. Buckingham: Open University Press.

Gott, M. and Hinchliff, S. (2004) Women's experiences of seeking treatment for sexual problems. Paper presented at the International, Interdisciplinary Conference on Gender, Sexuality and Health, Vancouver, 10–13 June.

Gott, M., Galena, E., Hinchliff, S. and Elford, H. (2004) "Opening a can of worms": GP and Practice Nurse barriers to talking about sexual health in primary care, *Family Practice* (21: 528–36).

Gott, M., Hinchliff, S. and Galena, E. (2004) A qualitative study to explore GP attitudes to discussing sexual health issues with older people, *Social Science and Medicine*, 58(11): 2093–103.

Greenhouse, P. (1995) A definition of sexual health, *British Medical Journal*, 310(6992): 1468–69.

Greer, G. (1991) *The Change: Women, Ageing and Menopause*. London: Hamish Hamilton.

Griffith, E. (1990) No sex please, we're over 60, *Nursing Times*, 84: 34–5.

Grossman, A.H. (1995) At risk, infected and invisible: older gay men and HIV/AIDS, *Journal of the Association of Nurses in AIDS Care*, 6(6): 13–19.

Gubrium, J.F. (1986) *Oldtimers and Alzheimer's: The Descriptive Organisation of Senility*. Greenwich, CT: JAI Press.

Gupta, K. (1990) Sexual dysfunction in elderly women, *Clinics in Geriatric Medicine*, 6(1): 197–203.

Gurland, M.J. and Gurland, R.V. (1980) Methods of research into sex and aging, in R. Green and J. Weiner (eds) *Methodology in Sex Research*. Washington, DC: Proceedings of the NIMH Conference, DHSS Publication Number (ADM) 80–766, Department of Health.

Guthrie, C. (1999) Nurses' perceptions of sexuality relating to patient care, *Journal of Clinical Nursing*, 8(3): 313–21.

Hacker, S.S. (1984) Students' questions about sexuality: implications for nurse educators, *Nurse Educator*, 9(4): 28–31.

Hajjar, R.R. and Kamel, H.K. (2003) Sex and the nursing home, *Clinics in Geriatric Medicine*, 19(3): 575–86.

Hart, G. and Wellings, K. (2002) Sexual behaviour and its medicalisation: in sickness and in health, *British Medical Journal*, 324: 896–900.

Hareven, T.K. (1977) Family time and historical time, *Daedalus*, 106(2): 57–70.

Hawkes, G. (1996) *A Sociology of Sex and Sexuality*. Buckingham and Philadelphia: Open University Press.

Health Protection Agency (HIV/STI Department, Communicable Disease Surveillance Centre) and the Scottish Centre for Infection and Environmental Health (2004) Unpublished Quarterly Surveillance Tables No 8, data until 12/03.

Heaphy, B., Yip, A. and Thompson, D. (2003) *Lesbian, Gay and Bisexual Lives Over 50*. Nottingham: York House Publications.

Heath, H. (1999) *Sexuality in Old Age*. London: NT Books.

Heath, H. and White, I. (2002) *The Challenge of Sexuality in Health Care*. Oxford: Blackwell Science Oxford.

Hellstrom, W.J.G. (ed.) (1999) *The Handbook of Sexual Dysfunction*. San Francisco: The American Society of Andrology.

Hendricks, J. and Hendricks, C.D. (1978) Sexuality in later life: an ageing population, in V. Carver and P. Liddiard (eds) *An Ageing Population*. London: Open University Press.

Hepworth, M. (1996) Consumer culture and social gerontology, *Education and Ageing*, 11(1): 19–30.

Hill, J., Bird, H. and Thorpe, R. (2003) Effect of rheumatoid arthritis on sexual activity and relationships, *Rheumatology*, 42: 280–6.

Hillman, J. (2000) *Clinical Perspectives on Elderly Sexuality*. Dordrecht: Kluwer Academic Publishers Group.

Hinchliff, S. and Gott, M. (2004) The meaning of sex in long term marriage, *Journal of Social and Personal Relationships (in press)*.

Hinchliff, S., Gott, M. and Galena, E. (2004a) A study of GPs' experiences of the gender-related barriers to discussing sexual health in primary care, *European Journal of General Practice*, 10: 56–60.

Hinchliff, S., Gott, M. and Galena, E. (2004b) Managing the sexual health needs of lesbian and gay patients in the primary care context: A qualitative study with General Practitioners. Paper presented at the 7th Congress of the European Federation of Sexology, Brighton, 12–14 May.

Hite, S. (1989) *The Hite Report: Nationwide Study of Female Sexuality*. New York: Dell Publishing Corps.

Hockey, J. and James, A. (1993) *Growing Up and Growing Old, Ageing and Dependency in the Life Course*. London: Sage.

Hodson, D. and Skeen, P. (1994) Sexuality and ageing: the hammerlock of myths, *The Journal of Applied Gerontology*, 13(3): 219–35.

Hogan, R. (1980) *Human Sexuality: A Nursing Perspective*. New York: Appleton-Century-Crofts.

Holgate, H.S. and Longman, C. (1998) Some peoples' psychological experiences of attending a sexual health clinic and having a sexually transmitted infection, *Journal of the Royal Society of Health*, 118(2): 94–6.

Hoolaghan, T. and Blache, G. (1993) *The Role of the GP in HIV Prevention: Health Promotion in General Practice Report*. London: Hampstead Health Promotions Department.

Hordern, A. (2000) Intimacy and sexuality for the woman with breast cancer, *Cancer Nursing*, 23(3): 230–6.

Hubbard, G., Cook, S., Tester, S. and Downs, M. (2003) *Sexual Expression in Institutional Care Settings for Older People*. CD produced by Department of Film and Media Studies, University of Stirling.

Humphrey, S. and Nazareth, I. (2001) GPs' views on their management of sexual dysfunction, *Family Practice*, 18(5): 516–18.

Information Services NHS Scotland (2003) Available online: http://www.isdscotland.org/isd/files/Gp%20Practice%20Staff-03xls (accessed 15 March 2004).

Jackson, S. and Scott, S. (1997) Gut reactions to matters of the heart: reflections on rationality, irrationality and sexuality, *The Sociological Review*, 45: 551–75.

James, O. (2003) The rise of the male, *The Observer*. http://observer.guardian.co.uk/magazine/story/0,11913,1041284,00.html (accessed 15 Apr. 2004).

Johnson, A.M. (1997) Studying sexual behaviour: what more do we need to know? *MRC News*, Autumn: 22–5.

Johnson, A.M., Mercer, C.H., Erens, B., Copas, A.J., McManus, S. and Wellings, K. et al. (2001) Sexual behaviour in Britain: partnerships, practices, and HIV risk behaviours, *The Lancet*, 358(9296): 1835–42.

Jones, R.L. (2002) "That's very rude, I shouldn't be telling you that": older women talking about sex, *Narrative Inquiry*, 12(1): 121–43.

Kaplan, H.S. (1995) *The Sexual Desire Disorders; Dysfunctional Regulation of Sexual Motivation*. New York: Brunner/Mazel.

Kaschak, E. and Tiefer, L. (2001) *A New View of Women's Sexual Problems*. Binghampton: The Haworth Press.

Katz, A. (2003) The "problem" is in the definition. http://bmj.bmjjournals.com/cgi/eletters/327/7412/426#36098 (accessed 25 May 2004).

Katz, S. (1996) *Disciplining Old Age: The Formation of Gerontological Knowledge*. Charlottesville, VA: The University Press of Virginia.

Katz, S. and Marshall, M. (2003) New sex for old: lifestyle, consumerism, and the ethics of aging well, *Journal of Aging Studies*, 17(1): 3–16.

Kaufmann, T. (1995) *HIV and AIDS and Older People*. London: Age Concern.

Kautz, D.D., Dickey, C.A and Stevens, M.N. (1990) Using research to identify why nurses do not meet established sexuality nursing care standards, *Journal of Nursing Quality Assurance*, 4(3): 69–78.

Keodt, A. (1974) The myth of the vaginal orgasm, in The Radical Therapy Collective (ed.) *The Radical Therapist*. Harmondsworth: Pelican.

Kessel, B. (2001) Sexuality in the older person, *Age and Ageing*, 30: 121–4.

Kilwein, J.H. (1989) No pain, no gain: a puritan legacy, *Health Education Quarterly*, 16: 9–12.

Kimmel, D.C. (1978) Adult development and aging: a gay perspective, *Journal of Social Issues*, 34: 113–30.

Kinsey, A.C., Pomeroy, W.B. and Martin, C.E. (1948) *Sexual Behavior in the Human Male*. Philadelphia, PA: W.B. Saunders.

Kinsey, A.C., Pomeroy, W.B., Martin, C.E. and Gebhard, P.H. (1953) *Sexual Behavior in the Human Female*. New York: W.B. Saunders.

Kleinschmidt, K.C (1997) Elder abuse: a review, *Annals of Emergency Medicine*, 30(4): 463–72.

Knight, I. (2003) Life in the old dogs yet, *Sunday Times News Review*, January 5: 4.

Kohiyar, G.A. (1983) Geriatric venereology, *Geriatric Medicine*, 13: 121–7.

Korpelainen, J.T., Pentti, N. and Myllyla, V.V. (1999) Sexual functioning among stroke patients and their spouses, *Stroke*, 39(4): 715–19.

Kubin, M., Wagner, G. and Fugl-Meyer, A.R. (2003) Epidemiology of erectile dysfunction, *International Journal of Impotence Research*, 15(1): 63–71.

Laner, J.A. (1978) Growing older male: heterosexual and homosexual, *Gerontologist*, 18: 496–501.

Larkin, P. (1974) *High Windows*. London: Faber and Faber.

LaTorre, A. and Kear, K. (1977) Attitudes towards sex in the aged, *Archives of Sexual Behavior*, 6(3): 203–13.

Laumann, E.O., Gagnon, J.H., Michael, R.T. and Michaels, S. (1994) *The Social Organization of Sexuality: Sexual Practices in the United States*. Chicago: University of Chicago Press.

Laumann, E.O., Paik, A. and Rosen, R. (1999) Sexual dysfunction in the United States: prevalence and predictors, *Journal of the American Medical Association*, 281(6): 537–44.

Lawler, J. (1991) *Behind the Screens: Nursing, Somology and the Problem of the Body*. Edinburgh: Churchill Livingstone.

Leenaars, P.E.M., Rombouts, R. and Kok, G. (1993) Seeking medical care for a sexually transmitted disease: determinants of delay-behaviour, *Psychology and Health*, 8: 17–32.

Leigh, B.C., Temple, M.T. and Trocki, K.F. (1993) The sexual behavior of US adults: results from a national survey, *American Journal of Public Health*, 83(10): 1400–8.

Levin, J. and Levin, W.C. (1980) *Ageism: Prejudice and Discrimination Against the Elderly*. Belmont, CA: Wadsworth.

Levin, S. (1987) Jane Fonda: from Barbarella to barbells, *Women's Sports and Fitness*, December.

Lewis, J. (1984) *Women in England 1870–1950*. London: Routledge.

Lewis, S. and Bor, R. (1994) Nurses' knowledge of and attitudes towards sexuality and the relationship of these with nursing practice, *Journal of Advanced Nursing*, 20(2): 251–9.

Ley, H., Morley, M. and Bramwell, R. (2002) The sexuality of a sample of older women: myths and realities explored, in: *Proceedings of the British Gerontology Society. Annual Conference*, Birmingham: British Society of Gerontology.

Loehr, J., Verma S. and Seguin, R. (1997) Issues of sexuality in older women, *Journal of Women's Health*, 6(4), 451–7.

Longstaff Mackay, J. (2001) 'Why have sex?', *British Medical Journal*, 322: 623.

Lupton, D. (1994) *Medicine as Culture: Illness, Disease and the Body in Western Societies*. London: Sage.

MacNab, F. (1994) *The Thirty Vital Years*. New York: Wiley and Sons.

Maddox, G. L. (ed.). (2001) *The Encyclopedia of Aging*, 3rd edn. New York: Springer.

Marr, J. (1994a) The impact of HIV on older people: part I, *Nursing Standard*, 8(46): 28–31.

Marr, J. (1994b) The impact of HIV on older people: part II, *Nursing Standard*, 8(47): 25–7.

Marshall, B. (2002), Hard science: gendered constructions of sexual dysfunction in the Viagra age, *Sexualities*, 5(2): 131–58.

Marsiglio, W. and Donnelly, D. (1991) Sexual relations in later life: a national study of married persons, *Journal of Gerontology*, 46(6): S338–S344.

Martin, C.E. (1981) Factors affecting sexual functioning in 60–79 year old married males, *Archives of Sexual Behaviour*, 10(5): 399–420.

Masters, W.H. and Johnson, V.E. (1966) *Human Sexual Response*. London: Churchill.

Masters, W.H and Johnson, V.E. (1970) *Human Sexual Inadequacy*. London: Churchill.

Matocho, L.K. and Waterhouse, J. (1993) Current nursing practice related to sexuality. *Researching in Nursing and Health*, 16, 371–8.

Matthias, R.E., Lubben, J.E., Atchison, K.A. and Schweitzer, S.O. (1997) Sexual activity and satisfaction among very old adults: results from a community-dwelling medicare population survey, *The Gerontologist*, 37(1): 6–14.

McCartney, J.R., Izeman, H., Rogers, D. and Cohen, N. (1987) Sexuality and the institutionalized elderly, *American Geriatric Journal Society*, 35(4): 331–3.

McDaniel, S. (1988) *Getting Older and Better: Women and Gender Assumptions in Canada's Aging Society*. Toronto: Butterworths.

McKee, K.J. (1998) The Body Drop: a framework for understanding recovery from falls in older people, *Generations Review*, 8: 11–12.

McKee, K.J. and Gott, M. (2002) Shame and the ageing body, in P. Gilbert and J. Miles (eds) *Understanding and Treating Body Shame*. London: Routledge.

McKinlay, J.B. and Feldman, H.A. (1994) Age-related variation in sexual activity and interest in normal men: results from the Massachusetts Male Aging Study, in A. Rossi (ed.) *Sexuality Across the Life Course: Proceedings of the MacArthur Foundation Research Network on Successful Mid-Life Development*. Chicago: University of Chicago Press.

McMullin, A. (2000) Diversity and the state of sociological aging theory, *Gerontologist*, 40(5): 517–30.

Meerabeau, L. (1999) The management of embarrassment and sexuality in health care, *Journal of Advanced Nursing*, 29(6): 1507–13.

Mercer, C.H., Fenton, K.A., Johnson, A.M. and Wellings, K. et al. (2003) Sexual function problems and help seeking behaviour in Britain: national probability sample survey, *British Medical Journal*, 327: 426–7.

Metters, J. (1998) Public to be quizzed about sex. http://news.bbc.co.uk/1/hi/health/203872.stm (accessed 16 Apr. 2004).

Michael, R.T., Wadsworth, J., Feinleib, J., Johnson, A.M., Laumann, E.O. and Wellings, K. (1998) Private sexual behaviour, public opinion, and public health policy related to sexually transmitted diseases: a US–British comparison. *American Journal of Public Health*, 88(5): 749–54.

Minkler, M. (1991) Gold in gray: reflections on business' discovery of the elderly market, in M. Minkler and C. Estes (eds) *Critical Perspectives on Aging: The Political and Moral Economy of Growing Old*. Amityville, NY: Baywood Publishing Company.

Moller, B. (2001) Porn calms Dutch seniors, staff say, *Globe and Mail*. http://www.walnet.org/csis/news/world_2001/gandm-01905.html (accessed 25 May 2004).

Montosiri, F., Salonia, A., Deho, F., Briganti, A. and Rigatti, P. (2002) The ageing male and erectile dysfunction, *World Journal Urolology*, 20: 28–35.

Mooradian, A.D. (1991) Geriatric sexuality and chronic diseases, *Clinics in Geriatric Medicine*, 7(1): 113–31.

Mooradian, A.D. and Greiff, V. (1990) Sexuality in older women, *Archives of Internal Medicine*, 150: 1033–38.

Moore, T.M., Strauss, J.L., Herman, S. and Donatucci, C.F. (2003) Erectile dysfunction in early, middle, and late adulthood: symptom patterns and psychosocial correlates, *Journal of Sex and Marital Therapy*, 29(5): 381–99.

Moynihan, R. (2003a) The making of a disease: female sexual dysfunction, *British Medical Journal*, 326: 45–7.

Monynihan, R. (2003b) Urologist recommends daily Viagra to prevent impotence, *British Medical Journal*, 326: 9.

Mulligan, T. and Moss, C.R. (1991) Sexuality and aging in male veterans: a cross sectional study of interest, ability and activity, *Archives of Sexual Behaviour*, 20(1): 17–25.

Mulligan, T. and Palguta, R.F. (1991) Sexual interest, activity, and satisfaction among male nursing home residents, *Archives of Sexual Behaviour*, 20(2): 199–204.

National Institute of Health (1992) *NIH Consensus Statement Online* 10(3): 1–31.

National Statistics (1998) *Key Health Statistics from General Practice*, Series MB6, No. 2. London: National Statistics.

National Statistics (2001) http://www.statistics.gov.uk/lib2001/viewerChart5229.html (accessed 20 Mar. 2004).

Nay, R. (1992) Sexuality and aged women in nursing homes, *Geriatric Nursing*, 13: 312–14.

Nazareth, I., Boynton, P. and King, M. (2003) Problems with sexual function in people attending London general practitioners: cross-sectional study, *British Medical Journal*, 327: 423–6.

Nelson, E.A. and Dannefer, D. (1992) Aged heterogeneity: fact or fiction? The fate of diversity in gerontological research, *The Gerontologist*, 32(1): 17–23.

Nichols, J.E., Speer, D.C. and Watson, B.J. et al. (2002) *Aging with HIV, Psychological, Social and Health Issue*. San Diego: Academic Press.

Nicolosi, A., Moreira, E.D., Jr. Shirai, M., Bin Mohd Tambi, M.I. and Glasser, D.B. (2003) Epidemiology of erectile dysfunction in four countries: cross-national study of the prevalence and correlates of erectile dysfunction, *Urology*, 61(1): 201–6.

Nicolson, P. (1993) Public values and private beliefs: why women refer themselves for sex therapy, in J.M. Ussher and C.D. Baker (eds) *Psychological Perspectives on Sexual Problems*. London: Routledge.

Nicolson, P. (1994) Anatomy and destiny, in P.Y.L. Choi and P. Nicolson (eds) *Female Sexuality: Psychology, Biology and Social Context*. Brighton: Harvester Wheatsheaf.

Nicolson, P. and Burr, J. (2003) What is 'normal' about women's (hetero)sexual desire and orgasm? A report of an in-depth interview study, *Social Science and Medicine*, 57(9): 1735–45.

Nieman, S. (2002) *Sexuality in Cancer and Palliative Care*, Social Work Monographs. Norwich: School of Social Work and Psychosocial Studies at the University of East Anglia.

NIH Consensus Development Panel on Impotence (1993) *American Medical Association*, 270: 83–90.

Nye, R.A. (1999) *Sexuality*. Oxford: Oxford University Press.

Öberg, P. (1996) The absent body: a social gerontological paradox, *Ageing and Society*, 16: 701–19.

Öberg, P. and Tornstam, L. (1999) Body images among men and women of different ages, *Ageing and Society*, 19(5): 629–44.

Ogden, G. (2001) Spiritual passion and compassion in late-life sexual relationships, *Electronic Journal of Human Sexuality*. http://www.ejhs.org/ volume4/Ogden.htm (accessed 25 May 2004).

Ogden, J. (2000) *Health Psychology*. Buckingham: Open University Press.

Opaneye, A.A. (1991) Sexuality and sexually transmitted diseases in older men attending the genito-urinary clinic in Birmingham, *Journal of the Royal Society of Health*, 111(1): 6–7.

OPCS (1991) 1991 Census statistics information obtained from 1990–1994: Supermap for Windows (professional edition, version 4,57c) Computer package. Space-Time Research, Hartwell, Australia.

Oxford English Dictionary (1989) http://www.oed.com/ (accessed 25 May 2003).

Pangman, V. and Seguire, M. (2000) Sexuality and the chronically ill older adult: a social justice issue, *Sexuality and Disability*, 18: 49–59.

Panser, L.A., Rhodes, T. and Girman, C.J. et al. (1995) Sexual function of men ages 40 to 79 years: the Olmstead County Study of urinary symptoms and health status among men, *Journal of American Geriatrics Society*, 43(10): 1107–11.

Park, K., Godstein, I., Andry, C., Siroky, M.B., Krane, R.J. and Azadzoi, K.M. (1997) Vasculogenic female sexual dysfunction: the hemodynamic basis for vaginal engorgement insufficiency and clitoral erectile insufficiency, *International Journal of Impotence Research*, 9: 27–37.

Parker, R.G. and Gagnon, J.H. (1995) *Conceiving Sexuality: Approaches to Sex Research in a Postmodern World*. New York and London: Routledge.

Payne, T. (1976) Sexuality of nurses: correlations of knowledge, attitudes and behaviour, *Nursing Research*, 25(4): 286–92.

Person, E.S. (1980) Sexuality as the mainstay of identity: psychoanalytic perspective, *Signs*, 5: 605–30.

Persson, G. (1980) Sexuality in a 70-year-old urban population, *Journal of Psychosomatic Research*, 24: 335–42.

Pfeiffer, E., Verdwoerdt, A. and Davis, G.C. (1972) Sexual behaviour in middle life, *The American Journal of Psychiatry*, 128(10): 82–7.

Phillipson, C. (1998) *Reconstructing Old Age*. London: Sage Publications.

Phillipson, C. (2002) Cultures of ageing: a debate. Paper presented at BSG conference, Birmingham, 12–14 September.

Plummer, K. (1975) *Sexual Stigma: An Interactionist Account*. London: Routledge and Kegan Paul.

Poindexter, C.C. and Linsk, N.L. (1999) "I'm just glad that I'm here". stories of seven African-American HIV-affected grandmothers, *Journal of Gerontological Social Work*, 32(1): 63–81.

Pointon, S. (1997) Myths and negative attitudes about sexuality in older people, *Generations Review*, 7(4): 6–8.

Positive Ageing Foundation of Australia A new mindset. http://www.positiveageing.com.au/PAFA_Research.htm (accessed 26 May 2004).

Potts, A., Gavey, N., Grace, V. and Vares, T. (2003) The downside of Viagra: women's experiences and concerns about Viagra use by men, *Sociology of Health and Illness*, 25(7): 697–719.

Potts, A., Grace, V., Gavey, N. and Vares, T. (2004) 'Viagra Stories': challenging 'erectile dysfunction', *Social Science and Medicine*, 59(3): 489–99.

Power, R. (2002) The application of qualitative research methods to the study of sexually transmitted infections, *Sexually Transmitted Infections*, 78: 87–9.

Read, S., King, M. and Watson, J. (1997) Sexual dysfunction in primary medical care: prevalence, characteristics and detection by the general practitioner, *Journal of Public Health Medicine*, 19(4): 387–91.

Reich, W. (1982) Function of the orgasm, in M. Brake (ed.), *Human Sexual Relations: A Reader*. Harmondsworth: Penguin.

Reinish, J. and Beasley, R. (1990) *The Kinsey Institute New Report on Sex: What You Must Know to Be Sexually Literate*. London: Penguin.

Reuben, D.R. (1970) *Everything You Ever Wanted to Know About Sex*. London and New York: W.H. Allen.

Richards, M. (2003) Yes, yes, yes! It's true – sex is good for you. http://www.handbag.com/relationships/sex/sexisgood/ (accessed 8 Sept. 2003).

Rickard, W. (1995) HIV/AIDS and older people, *Generations Review*, 5(3): 2–6.

Rimm, E. (2003) Exercise may prolong men's sex lives, *MSNBC News*.http://msnbc.msn.com/id/3077047/ (accessed 15 Apr. 2004).

Ringheim, K. (1995) Ethical issues in social science research with special reference to sexual behaviour research, *Social Science and Medicine*, 40(12): 1691–7.

Ritchie, J. and Spencer, L. (1994) Qualitative data analysis for applied policy research, in A. Bryman and R.G. Burgess (eds), *Analyzing Qualitative Data*. London: Routledge.

Roddick, S. (2002) Quoted in L. Brooks, 'Lights, camera, phwoar', *The Guardian*. http://www.guardian.co.uk/gs/story/0,2604,821123,00.html (accessed 2 Jan. 2003).

Rogstad, K.E. and Bignell, C.J. (1991) Age is no bar to sexually acquired infection, *Age and Ageing*, 20: 377–8.

Rosenfeld, D. (1999) Identity work among lesbian and gay elderly, *Journal of Aging Studies*, 13: 121–44.

Rotosky, S.S. and Brown Travis, C. (2000) Menopause and sexuality: ageism and sexism unite, in C. Brown Travis and J.W. White (eds) *Sexuality, Society and Feminism*. Washington, DC: American Psychological Association.

Royal College of General Practitioners (1995) Foreword in H. Curtis, T. Hoolaghan, and C. Jewitt (eds) *Sexual Health in General Practice*. Abingdon and New York: Radcliffe Medical Press.

Sahai, V. and Demeyere, P. (1996) Sexual health: are we targeting the right age groups?, *Canadian Journal of Public Health*, 87(1): 40–1.

Sarkadi, A. and Rosenqvist, U. (2001) Contradictions in the medical encounter: female sexual dysfunction in primary care contacts, *Family Practice*, 18: 161–6.

Schiavi, R. (1999) *Aging and Male Sexuality*. Cambridge: Cambridge University Press.

Schlesinger, B. (1996) The sexless years or sex rediscovered, *Journal of Gerontological Social Work*, 26: 117–31.

Schofield, M. (1965) *The Sexual Behaviour of Young People*. Harmondsworth: Penguin.

Scoular, A., Duncan, B. and Hart, G. (2001) "That's the sort of place ... where filthy men go ...": a qualitative study of women's perceptions of genitourinary medicine services, *Sexually Transmitted Infections*, 77: 340–43.

Sherman, B. (1999) *Sex, Intimacy, and Aged Care*. London: Jessica Kingsley Publishers.

Ship, J.A., Wolff, A. and Selik, R.M. (1991) Epidemiology of acquired immune deficiency syndrome in persons aged 50 years or older, *Journal of Acquired Immune Deficiencies Syndromes*, 4: 84–8.

Simons, J.S. and Carey, M.P. (2001) Prevalence of sexual dysfunctions: results from a decade of research, *Archives of Sexual Behaviour*, 30(2): 177–219.

Skelton, J.R. and Matthews, P.M. (2001) Teaching sexual history: talking to health care professionals in primary care, *Medical Education*, 35: 603–8.

Skevington, S.M. (1999) Measuring quality of life in Britain: introducing the WHOQOL-100, *Journal of Psychosomatic Research*, 47(5): 449–59.

Skoog, J. (1996) Sex and Swedish 85-year olds, *The New England Journal of Medicine*, 334(17): 1140–41.

Smith-Rosenberg, C. (1985) *Disorderly Conduct: Visions of Gender in Victorian America*. New York: Oxford University Press.

Sontag, S. (1978) The double standard of ageing, in V. Carver and P. Liddiard (eds) *An Ageing Population*. Milton Keynes: Open University Press.

Sontag, S. (1979) *The Double Standard of Aging*, New York: Farrar, Straus and Giroux. Available online at http://www.mediawatch.com/sontag.html (accessed 16 May 2004).

Sontag, S. (1991) *Illness as Metaphors and AIDS and its Metaphors*. London: Penguin Books.

Spector, I.P. and Fremeth, S.M. (1996) Sexual behaviors and attitudes of geriatric residents in long-term care facilities, *Journal of Sex and Marital Therapy*, 22(4): 235–46.

Stall, R. and Catania, J. (1994) AIDS risk behaviors among late middle-aged and elderly Americans: the national AIDS behavioral surveys, *Archives of Internal Medicine*, 154: 57–63.

Starr, B.D. and Weiner, M.B. (1982) *The Starr-Weiner Report on Sex and Sexuality in the Mature Years*. New York: McGraw-Hill.

Steinke, E.E. (1994) Knowledge and attitudes of older adults about sexuality in ageing: a comparison of two studies, *Journal of Advanced Nursing*, 19: 477–85.

Stuart, G. and Sundeen, S. (1979) *Principles and Practice of Psychiatric Nursing*. St Louis, MO: Mosby.

Stokes, T. and Mears, J. (2000) Sexual health and the practice nurse: a survey of reported practice and attitudes, *The British Journal of Family Planning*, 26(2): 89–92.

Sullivan, C. (2003) The butt stops here, *The Guardian*, 19 November. http://www.guardian.co.uk/comment/story/0,3604,1088189,00.html (accessed 15 Apr. 2004).

Tate, P. (2000) Sex-lives and videotape: sexual history taking in primary care, *Family Practice*, 17(1): 100.

Tellier, T. (2003) *The Livia Stoke Foundation Annual Report 2002/2003*. Edmonton: Livia Stoke Foundation.

Thomas, F. (1991) Correlates of sexual interest among elderly men, *Psychological Reports*, 68: 620–2.

Tiefer, L. (1986) In pursuit of the perfect penis: the medicalization of male sexuality, *American Behavioral Scientist*, 29: 579–99.

Tiefer, L. (1995) *Sex is Not a Natural Act*. Boulder, CO: Westview Press.

Tiefer, L. (2000) The social construction and social effects of sex research: the sexological model of sexuality, in C. Brown Travis and J.W. White (eds) *Sexuality, Society and Feminism*. Washington, DC: American Psychological Association.

Tiefer, L. (2001) Arriving at a 'new view' of woman's sexual problems: background, theory and activism, in E. Kaschak and L. Tiefer (eds) *A New View of Women's Sexual Problems*. New York, London and Oxford: The Haworth Press, Inc.

Tiefer, L. and Giami, A. (2002) Sexual behaviour and its medicalisation, Letter, *British Medical Journal*, 325: 45.

Tomlinson, J. and Wright, D. (2004) Impact of erectile dysfunction and its subsequent treatment with sildenafil: qualitative study, *British Medical Journal*, 328: 1037–40.

Townsend, P. (1981) The structured dependency of the elderly: the creation of social policy in the twentieth century, *Ageing and Society*, 1(1): 5–28.

Travis, C.B., Meginis, K.L. and Bardari, K.M. (2000) Beauty, sexuality, and identity: the social control of women, in C. Brown Travis and J.W. White (eds) *Sexuality, Society and Feminism*. Washington, DC: American Psychological Association.

Tunaley, J.R. (1995) Body size, food and women's identity: a qualitative psychological study across the life span. University of Sheffield. Unpublished PhD thesis.

Tunaley, J.R., Walsh, S. and Nicolson, P. (1999) 'I'm not bad for my age': the meaning of body size and eating in the lives of older women, *Ageing and Society*, 19(6): 741–59.

Turnbull, A. (2002) *Opening Doors: A Literature Review*. London: Age Concern.

Turner, B.S. (1984) *The Body and Society: Explorations in Social Theory*. London: Sage.

UNAIDS (2002) Impact of AIDS on older populations. http://www.unaids.org/en/in+focus/topic+areas/older+people.asp (accessed 25 May 2004).

Vance, C.S. (1989) *Pleasure and Danger: Exploring Female Sexuality*. London: Pandora Press.

Van der Geest, S. (2001) "No strength": sex and old age in a rural town in Ghana, *Social Science and Medicine*, 53: 1383–96.

Verhoeven, V., Bovijn, K., Helder, A., Peremans, L., Hermann, I., Van Royen, P., Denekens, J. and Avonts, D. (2003) Discussing STIs: doctors are from Mars, patients from Venus, *Family Practice*, 20: 11–15.

Verwoerdt, A., Pfeiffer, E. and Wang, H. (1969) Sexual behavior in senescence: changes in sexual activity and interest in aging men and women, *Journal of Geriatric Psychiatry*, 2: 163–80.

Victor, C. (1991) *Health and Health Care in Later Life*. Buckingham: Open University Press.

Vincent, C. (2002) Health challenges for older women: some implications for sexual health, *Sexual and Relationship Therapy*, 17(3): 241–52.

von Krafft-Ebing, R. (1886) *Psychopathia Sexualis: With Especial Reference to Contrary Sexual Instincts, a Medico-legal Study*. Trans. C.G., Chaddock (1918), Philadelphia, PA: F.A. Davis Co.

Walker, A. (1986) Pensions and the production of poverty in old age, in A. Walker and C. Phillipson (eds) *Ageing and Social Policy*. Aldershot: Gower.

Wallace, M. (2003) Sexuality and aging in long-term care, *Annals of Long Term Care*, 11(2): 53–9.

Wall-Haas, C.L. (1991) Nurses' attitudes towards sexuality in adolescent patients, *Paediatric Nursing*, 17(6): 549–55.

Waterhouse, J. and Metcalfe, M. (1991) Attitudes towards nurses discussing sexual concerns with patients, *Journal of Advanced Nursing*, 16: 1048–54.

Webb, C. (1988) A study of nurses' knowledge and attitudes about sexuality in health care, *International Journal of Nursing Studies*, 25(3): 235–44.

Webb, C. and Cordingley, L. (1999) Expressing sexuality, in S.J. Redfern and F.M. Ross (eds) *Nursing Older People*, 3rd edn. Edinburgh: Churchill Livingstone.

Weeks, D. (2003) Sex is good for you. www.handbag.com/relationships/sex/sexis-good/ (accessed 18 May 2004).

Weeks, J. (1985) *Sexuality and its Discontents: Meanings, Myths and Modern Sexualities*. London: Routledge and Kegan Paul.

Weeks, J. (1986) *Sexuality*. London and New York: Routledge.

Weeks, J. (1989) *Sex, Politics and Society: The Regulation of Sexuality Since 1800*, 2nd edn. Harlow: Pearson Education Group Limited.

Weg, R.B (ed.) (1983) *Sexuality in the Later Years: Roles and Behaviours*. New York: Academic Press.

Weil, L. (2001). Reissue. In the service of truth: remembering Barbara MacDonald, in B. MacDonald and C. Rich (eds) *Look Me in the Eye*. Denver, Co: Spinsters Ink Books.

Wellings, K., Field, J., Johnson, A.M. and Wadsworth, J. (1994) *Sexual Behaviour in Britain: The National Survey of Sexual Attitudes and Lifestyles*. London: Penguin.

Westlake, C., Dracup, K., Wladen, J.A. and Fonarow, G. (1999) Sexuality of patients with advanced heart failure and their spouses or partners, *The Journal of Heart and Lung Transplantation*, 18(11):1133–8.

Weston, A. (1993) Challenging assumptions, *Nursing Times*, 89: 18–26.

White, C.B and Catania, J.A. (1982) Psychoeducational intervention for sexuality with the aged, family members of the aged and people who work with the aged, *International Journal of Aging and Human Development*, 15: 121–38.

White, I. (1994) Nurses' social construction of sexuality within a cancer care context: an exploratory case study. Unpublished MSc thesis, City University, London.

Widdus, R., Meheus, A. and Short, R. (1990) The management of risk in sexually transmitted diseases, *Daedalus*, 119: 177–91.

Wiley, D. and Bortz, W.M. (1996) Sexuality and aging – usual and successful, *Journals of Gerontology*, 51A(3): M142–M146.

Willcocks, D., Peace, S. and Kellaher, L. (1987) *Private Lives in Public Places: A Research Based Critique of Residential Life in Local Authority Old People's Homes*. London: Tavistock.

Willcocks, D., Peace, S., Kellaher, L. and Ring, A. (1982) *The Residential Life of Old People: A Study of 100 Local Authority Homes*. London: 12(1) Survey Research Unit, Polytechnic of North London.

Wilson, M.E. and Williams, H.A. (1988) Oncology nurses' attitudes and behaviours related to sexuality of patients with cancer, *Oncology Nursing Forum*, 15: 49–52.

The Working Group for a New View of Women's Sexual Problems (2001), in E. Kaschak and L. Teifer (eds) *A New View of Women's Sexual Problems*. Binghampton, NY: The Haworth Press.

World Health Organization (2001) Gender and reproductive rights: sexual health. http://www.who.int/reproductive-health/gender/sexualhealth.html (accessed 23 Oct. 2003).

Youdell, D., Warwick, I. and Whitty, G. (1995) *Someone to talk to: HIV, AIDS and People Over 50*. London: Age Concern.

Zilbergeld, B. (1992) *The New Male Sexuality: The Truth about Men, Sex and Pleasure*. New York: Bantam.

Zingmond, D.S., Wenger, N.S., Crystal, S. et al. (2002) Circumstances at HIV diagnosis and progression of disease in older HIV-infected Americans, *American Journal of Public Health*, 91(7): 1117–20.

Index